Un-Broken Children

Removing Labels Restoring Health & Wellness

Mary M Ernsberger, CHN, MS, M.Ed.

For more information, or to book an event, contact:

https://mountainfamilyholisticnutrition.com

ISBN-13: 978-1508847649
ISBN-10: 1508847649

Book design by: Mary M Ernsberger
Cover design by: KDP Publications

Library of Congress Control Number: 2018675309
Printed in the United States of America

Acknowledgments

I would like to thank God – The Universal Source – Creator – Higher Power – for allowing me this opportunity and free will to experience life. Each experience has been another paving stone in my life's path that has led me to where I am today.

I would also like to thank K.C. Miller, Linda Bennett, Caroline Frasier and all the other teachers and students I have shared classes with at the Southwest Institute of Healing Arts in Tempe, AZ as well as the instructors at the American College of Healthcare Sciences. You have all inspired me to recognize the greatness in others, and to finally recognize the greatness in myself. Without that gift, I would not have had the courage to undertake this project.

I pray that – through this book – we, as a society, will endeavor to stop the derogatory labeling of every person we perceive as different. May we instead bless and acknowledge that difference and honor that person for the light and knowledge he or she adds to our lives in their own unique way.

Table of Contents

Introduction

When children fail to fit into the little box society calls "normal" the search begins to identify what is wrong with them. A wide range of labels have been created to describe these BROKEN children. A natural following to being diagnosed with a disorder is the little pill that will make these children appear normal - that will help them fit back into that little box

I disagree. No child is broken. They have their own special genius within that is being kept hidden. It is time to unlock these boxes and let these children shine. It begins here.

The intent of this book is three fold.

First - to educate on and explore the various mental, emotional, behavioral, and learning disorders that children are most often diagnosed with, along with the symptoms used to reach the diagnosis and the tools the medical community uses to identify which disorder you or your child has.

Second – to awaken to the over diagnosis and drugging that often accompanies these disorders, evaluate the multitude of pharmaceutical drugs currently prescribed to treat the symptoms along with the potential dangerous side effects and contraindications for their use.

Third – to examine the importance of nutrition as it relates to learning, the use of natural therapies as a compliment to or a replacement for pharmaceutical therapies, theories on how we learn, and the unique way the brain processes, stores and replays learned information.

It is believed, by many in the holistic and complementary/alternative medicine (CAM) field, that by taking the time to discover the root or core issue of the behavior or symptom and honoring the body by restoring balance on a physical, mental, emotional and spiritual level, we can avoid the over diagnosis and in turn the drugging of future generations.

In addition, I want parents to know that they are never alone in the struggle to allowing your child to be the authentic individual and express the unique genius they were born with. Check around your local area for support or networking groups, i.e., MeetUp.com; and/or alternative therapy practitioners, i.e., naturopaths, herbalists, and nutritionists. These groups and individuals are out there waiting to help you, to support you, as you meet your needs and those of your family. If you are unable to find a group, talk with a natural therapy practitioner and ask them to consider facilitating a group, especially if you know of other families with young people who are going through the same thing.

There are many internet sites available to make the search faster and easier, however, it is important to remember to verify the source of the information online. In other words, avoid using Wikipedia. Though they do have some valuable information, the fact that anyone can update or add information to a listing makes it one of the least reliable sources for verifiable information. If you are interested in learning more about natural remedies, look for a website sponsored by an individual that has the education and experience behind him/her, instead of someone who is simply regurgitating what they have read from somewhere else.

If you want to explore the information available on brain-based learning or learning styles/multiple intelligences (MI), find sources that have been involved in the research in these areas. I am actually including some online resources for FREE MI evaluations for both you and your child in this book. This will provide you with the opportunity to see where you and your child are alike in your learning capabilities – but more important, it will provide you with an opportunity to celebrate your differences. You may be surprised at the results.

As you read, and (more importantly) after you are finished, I challenge you to look past the labels. Stand up and say **ENOUGH!** Our children are the future of our country and our world and they deserve better. Kids – Stand Up for Yourself. You are worthy – You have a genius spark within you. You decide how bright that spark can become – BUT – You must take responsibility for how you are perceived. Like Attracts Like. If you want to be taken seriously when you speak – If you want respect – If you want to be heard – You must hear, respect, and take others seriously. Let go of the assumptions. It must be a team effort. Change is rarely easy – but it is so worth it. Are you ready to accept the challenge?

LEGAL DISCLAIMER: The statements in this book are the opinion of the author based on her education and research and have not been evaluated by the Food and Drug Administration. They are not intended to diagnose, treat, cure, or prevent any disease. Before you make changes based on the information provided, check with your primary care physician or other medical advisor.

Chapter 1

How It All Began

Any single parent can tell you that raising a child, or in my case children, on your own is no piece of cake. You are the mom and the dad (or the dad and the mom), even if the other parent is in the picture, you are the one who is there on a full-time basis always trying to balance your time, work, and of course money, and hoping that each child knows how much you love them and that all that you do is truly for them. Now throw in one of any number of diagnoses of childhood emotional, behavioral, or learning disorder. Soon to follow are the resulting calls from the school and disruptions at home. The need for support, honest information and options can be overwhelming.

Some single parents are lucky enough to have a support system that comes from family and friends. Others are on their own – like I was. Both of my parents died before I had my children. I was adopted, as a baby, and I had no idea who or if I still had a biological family out there. I have a brother, who was also adopted. He lived in another state, and we had never been that close. Either way, finding ways to meet those needs is an ongoing search.

I have decided to share my story because I want other parents to know they are not alone. I believe that most single parents would much rather receive encouragement from those around them than the pity single parents are often offered. I know I did and still do. Whether you realize it at the time, all of us are living the daily choices we make. To support those choices, we are looking for options and people who are willing to stand with us, at least I was. When I divorced my husband of just over eight years, my youngest son was just over a year old. I had been feeling like I was already a single parent, raising four children instead of the three I had at home. He was an over the road trucker and I hated the idea that I had to keep reminding him that he had a family at home that really needed his support physically, emotionally, and financially. When I pressed him to choose between his family and his truck, it really hurt when he chose the truck.

It has taken many, many years for me to stop blaming myself. Have you ever done that? It must be my fault. It was never anything he did. What is wrong with me? So instead, I buried those feelings, put on my "I have everything under control" mask, and went about doing what I needed to do to keep a roof over my children's heads, clothes on their backs, and food in their tummies. Have you ever felt like there were two people vying for control of your life, or that there were two people sharing your mind and body? For me, this goes back to when I was much younger. Personal self-esteem was never my strong suit.

Now work self-esteem; that was a different matter. I loved to be challenged. Tell me a chore was impossible, just sit back and watch me do it. I felt like one person when I was at work, a totally different person when I was at home and both of these people were stuck on a hamster's wheel, going round and round. Or maybe I had taken Bill Murray's place in the movie Groundhog Day. Every day was a carbon copy of the day before. I never gave another thought to having a personal life, I believed, at that time, that I was unable to choose a man who would be an honest and responsible choice and I was sure no one would want a single mom with three little kids.

So, each day it was get up, get ready, get the kids up, dressed, fed and out the door to the sitter or to school so I could go to work. After work, the routine continued, pick up the kids, go home, fix dinner (unless I went through a local fast-food drive thru), help the older two with homework, then it is bath time, jammies on, read a story and nighty-night. Wow, now I can breathe. Days turned into years and before I knew it, my youngest son was finally old enough to go to Head Start and the next year, he would be in kindergarten.

It is true when people say, "Don't blink" because one moment they are just learning to crawl or walk and the next moment they are waving at you from the window of the school bus. What happened? Where did the time go?

Chapter 2

The First Diagnosis

The problems began with a late afternoon phone call from the Aurora Police Department. The officer said my son had apparently wondered away from the Head Start center and they had been called in. Before I could totally freak out, the officer assured me that he had been found and was doing fine. I told her I was on my way.

When I arrived at the center, I was immediately greeted by the head teacher. Honestly, I had no desire to talk to her until I saw my son and made sure he was ok. She began apologizing profusely, repeatedly saying that this had never happened before, and actually trying to take the responsibility off her staff and placing it on a five year old little boy. Ok, so yes, I know my son made a really bad decision but in this case, could I really place all the blame on his actions? I supposed I could say he was to blame for separating himself from the rest of his class and his teacher. But how could they be unaware that they were short a child? How had this much time passed before they even noticed? Nick, my youngest son, was just 5 years old, and no matter how many times she apologized, I was absolutely livid. Nick came running over and I could see he was fine.

A new center had recently been built and was complete except for the playground area. The lead teacher explained that a classroom teacher would load the kids on a bus and take them to the old center's location, letting the kids play outside for an hour or so and then put them back on the bus and bring them back to the new center. Today, after being taken to the old school, my son had apparently decided he wanted to continue playing after the teacher told them it was time to get back on the bus. She said that Nick had originally followed the teacher's directions, along with the rest of the children, sitting in the front seat, right by the bus door. She went on to explain that the driver and teacher began counting the children. And, she thought, as soon as the driver and teacher walked past him, Nick slipped back out the open bus door and hid behind a bush next to the playground until the bus left.

I never found out how much time had actually lapsed before they realized Nick was missing. There are almost 2 miles between the old center and the new location. But considering the distance, it must have been quite a while before they even noticed. According to the lead teacher, the bus had driven back to the center, all the kids had been unloaded, and the next activity had begun before any of the teachers finally noticed they were one child short.

In the meantime, Nick had apparently played at the old center until he got bored being all alone and decided he needed to return to the center. He had walked about a mile or so up the road, crossed a major intersection – twice – and ended up in the parking lot of a closed gas station.

The lead teacher said that the school had called the police as soon as they noticed a child was missing. The young female officer I spoke to told me she had heard the report of a missing little boy, about the same time as a report came in of a small child walking up the roadway by himself. She said she saw several cars in the parking lot of a closed gas station on the corner of a main intersection, so she pulled in. She told me that when she exited the car, she saw the "cutest little blonde haired boy standing there holding a rock and telling several adults, who had gotten out of their cars, to get away." The officer said one of the adults told her that she had called the police as she followed the little boy up the roadway, worried that he was going to get hit by a car. She said she rolled down her window and offered him a ride, but he refused and told her he knew where he was going. She told the officer that she was a mother, and she would hope someone would look after her child if he ever got himself in this type of situation.

The officer said she sent the crowd away as she approached the little boy and asked him his name and what he was doing out there all by himself. She said the boy told her his name was Nick and he was on the way to his school. She said she told him his teacher was worried about him and asked if she could give him a ride. She said, Nick told her that his mom had always told him to never get in a car with a stranger – that is why he had the rock – but since she was a police officer, he knew she would be ok.

The officer said Nick walked around to the passenger side door, opened it, and got in. After latching his own seat belt, he told the officer he would give her directions to his school. As the police car got closer to the Head Start center, Nick pointed out the red roof and told her where she needed to turn.

I sat down by Nick and asked him how he knew which way to go. With that wonderful "DUH" expression that little kids give, he said he had watched what roads the bus took when it brought him there. I know he could tell how worried I was, and he promised he would never do anything like that again.

He went on to explain what he had done and how he got to where the police office picked him up. He admitted he got off the bus and hid behind inside a play spaceship. He said he waited for the bus to leave and then went back to the swings. He said he thought it would be more fun having the whole playground to himself, but he said it was actually boring without the other kids, so he decided he needed to get back to school.

Nick said he left the playground and closed and locked the gate like he had seen his teacher do. He said he started walking down the street. He was very proud of the fact that he stayed on the side of the road and on the sidewalks where possible. He also said some strangers in cars had pulled over and tried to give him a ride, but he threw rocks at them and told them to go away. With those big blue eyes, Nick said he gave the police officer directions to make sure she could find her way.

As a parent, we all wonder how many of the things we try to teach our children actually sink in. I was torn between the anger I felt from the fear for his safety and the pride I felt that he knew where to go and to never get into a car with a stranger. Most of all, I just wanted to hug him and hold on for a long time. Then reality set in. This was one really smart kid – what was I in for as he got older?

Living in rural Missouri, every place you go, you have to drive. The school was about 15 miles from where I worked and it would take anywhere from 20-25 minutes, depending on traffic, to get there to pick Nick up after work. One of the teachers told me they were opening up another Head Start in the same town I worked in.

I went up to the new location and spoke to the head teacher. I felt comfortable that Nick would like these new surroundings, plus it would be a lot easier to pick him up since my work was only about a mile away. I asked about transferring to the new location. Nick seemed a bit leery about the new center. I tried to explain the travel time and how much easier it was to be close to him. Nick, always the agreeable child, said everything would be ok. Nick's the type of child that no matter how bad a day he has, by the time the next morning rolled around, he had forgiven and forgotten and was ready to start again. I often wish my other two children were so even tempered.

A few months passed and I began noticing a change in Nick's behavior. When asked, he told me that school was boring. I spoke to the teacher in Nick's room and asked her if the kids were being taught their letters and how to print their names. I explained that Nick would be entering kindergarten in August and I would really appreciate it if they would work with him. The teacher's reply surprised me. She said, "If he tells us he wants to learn how to write his name, we will help him." I asked her why they would ask a 5 year old what he wanted to learn, instead of providing a structured environment to promote learning. I also said that I thought that the purpose of Head Start was to provide children with a "head start" before they entered regular school. The teacher said they encourage the children to make their own decisions instead of telling them what to do.

After the playground incident, I knew Nick was smart but because he was only five (5) years old, I struggled trying to wrap my brain around him having the ability to make what I considered "grown up" decisions regarding his learning environment. I decided to go to the lead teacher and was extremely disappointed in her response. She echoed the class teacher and told me if I was unhappy with the way they did things; I could always take my son out of this school and put him somewhere else. I felt like I was being put between a rock and a hard place. The teacher knew I was a single mom and needed a school setting that was close to work. I wanted safe place for my son to stay while I worked. I wanted an environment that nurtured a love of education and encouraged the kids to have independent thoughts, which he seemed to get at the other center. But, if I transferred him back to the old center, I would risk being late picking him up each evening. Then there were the late fees. The school charged $10.00 for the first five minutes and then $1.00 per minute after that when a parent was late. If you have ever worked a job where you went from paycheck to paycheck just trying to make ends meet, you know that every dollar counts.

A couple of weeks later, the lead teacher asked to talk to me. She said that a county psychologist made regular visits to the daycare and one of the teachers had raised concerns that there might be something wrong with my son. That was the first time I had ever heard of Attention Deficit Hyperactivity Disorder (ADHD). She said I needed to make an appointment with the psychologist for an evaluation.

I made the appointment and when we arrived, Nick said hi to the psychologist and went right to playing with the toys in the office. Against one wall I saw five or six plastic bins with different toys in each one. The psychologist sat down next to me and began telling me what an enjoyable son I had. She said he was very bright but seemed to have trouble completing projects. I reminded her that he was only 5 and wondered why that was a problem. I told her that he often sat for an hour or more, engrossed in play both alone and with other kids. After spending maybe, a total of 15 minutes with this psychologist, she announced that he 'definitely had ADHD". She wrote out a prescription for Ritalin and told me my son needed to take this medication to control his behavior. I pressed her for an explanation for at least one specific example that she had observed that led her to this conclusion. She stated that upon our arrival, he should have walked over to the multi-colored bins of toys, selected one, and sat down to play. I asked her how he was supposed to know what toy he wanted to play with if he failed to explore what toys were available. I told her the fact that he had gone from bin to bin checking out the different toys showed me his level of curiosity. I asked her to explain why curiosity was wrong in a child. She failed to respond so I asked her if she had children of her own. She became defensive telling me, 'No', but that had nothing to do with her ability to diagnose a child.

The next day, I asked the lead teacher to tell me why she had referred Nick to the psychologist. She said the psychologist came into the center on a regular basis and conducted "play therapy" with some of their students. She said Nick had not been specifically referred to the psychologist. I asked if he had not specifically been referred, why was I told to make an appointment? I told her I had no desire to drug my child as I saw him as a normal five (5) year old who was naturally curious. She stated that if he had been prescribed medication for a diagnosed condition, and I refused to give him the medication, they would have no choice but to make him leave the center.

As you can imagine, that left me with a real problem. I have two people telling me my son needs to take these drugs and neither one can give me a clear explanation as to why. I had no idea what to do. Luckily, it was a Friday, and I decided it would be better to avoid making a snap decision. I would have the weekend to think it over. I really hoped that something would happen or I would meet someone that would clear up some of my questions. Nick seemed like a perfectly happy, energetic five-year-old little boy. He never threw fits or broke things. If anything, he was a bit clingy.

Saturday night I was lying in bed and listening to a talk radio show (that I just happened to turn into). The host of the show, Art Bell, was interviewing an attorney that represented people on health related legal issues. I decided to call in and see if I could get some help. Surprisingly, I got through the switchboard and spoke to the attorney. After telling him my story, he told me that Head Start was a Federal Government Program and as long as I qualified financially, they had no right to force my son out of the center. He advised me to find an attorney in my state if they continued to press the issue. He told me this was a continuing and growing problem in the public school system. I asked why a school would press the issue of giving medications to little children. The attorney told me that back in 1991 that the Federal Government had passed a bill that allowed school districts to apply for federal funding based on the number of children that were in their "learning disability" classes.

So, I had my answer, it was all about the money, not my child and what was best for him. Even more important, I learned that there are some people out there that are willing to exploit their position of power to get you to do what they want. I honestly would never have doubted that she had the ability to force my son out of the program if I had missed that radio show and had never spoken with that attorney.

Feeling empowered, I returned to the center on Monday and advised the staff that I had no plans to medicate my child. Again, I was told that without medication, my son would be unable to continue attending Head Start. I told the lead teacher that I had spoken to an attorney, and I knew that because Head Start was a federally funded program, they had no authority to force him out. Following my chat with the lead teacher, Nick remained at Head Start for the remaining two or three months until he started kindergarten. None of the teachers had anything else to say about ADHD or the medications. Kindergarten and first grade were actually very uneventful in the Verona School District and Attention Deficit Hyperactivity Disorder was never mentioned.

If any school official threatens to remove your child from school because you refuse to medicate your child, copy and paste the following Federal law and give them a copy.

Title 20 of United States Code:
Chapter 33, Subchapter II,

ASSISTANCE FOR EDUCATION OF ALL CHILDREN WITH DISABILITIES

§ 1412, State Eligibility

(25) Prohibition on mandatory medication

(A) In general,

The State educational agency shall prohibit State and local educational agency personnel from requiring a child to obtain a prescription for a substance covered by the Controlled Substances Act as a condition of attending school, receiving an evaluation under subsection (a) or (c) of section 1414 of this title, or receiving services under this chapter.

(B) Rule of construction

Nothing in subparagraph (A) shall be construed to create a Federal prohibition against teachers and other school personnel consulting or sharing classroom-based observations with parents or guardians regarding a student's academic and functional performance, or behavior in the classroom or school, or regarding the need for evaluation for special education or related services under paragraph (3).

In April of 2001, with only two months of the school year left, we moved to Arizona. It was quite an adjustment. The school in Missouri was small – less than 1000 students in grades K-12 - and many of the kids had or would go from class to class, year to year, through all 12 grades, with the same kids they had gone to kindergarten with. In Arizona, the elementary school the boys attended had over 600 kids in grades K-5. My other two children had no problem integrating into the new school, but my youngest son was overwhelmed. The classes back in Missouri were small enough that the kids were used to openly sharing in class. In Arizona, it was strictly forbidden in this new school environment. Nick openly showed how overwhelmed he felt with that many students and all the new rules. I attempted to calm his fears and fully expected that since there was only six or seven weeks of school left – before summer break – it would be smooth sailing. I had no idea know how rough the waters would be.

It turns out the biggest adjustment for Nick was when it came time for recess. Back in those days, he was very friendly, sometimes to the point that it overwhelmed the children around him. He would walk up to anyone and just assume his attention was welcome. But then we are talking about 15-20 kids at a time at his old school. Here, in the three first grade classes, there were around 90 kids, and all of them would be on the playground with only three or four teachers to keep an eye on all of them.

The Mesa Public School System used what was called the "Step Discipline Plan" which consisted of four steps. Step 1 was time-out for about 5 minutes. If the child stood quietly, they could return to their table or desk when their time was up. If the child was unable to do that, they were put into Step 2, which added another 5 minutes to time out. So now the child has to stand in one place, face the wall without turning around or making any sound for 10 minutes. If the child was unable to complete their 10 minutes of time out, they are put into Step 3. In Step 3, the child was removed from the classroom and taken to the counselor or principal's office. Once there, they are talked to, asked to explain what they did wrong and basically say they would never do it again, the child was then allowed to return to the classroom. If the offense is severe enough, the child is placed in Step 4. At least once and sometimes twice a week, I was being called to the school and told that Nick had been in "Steps" today.

Many of the things I got called about seemed petty, or almost ridiculous, especially considering the ages of the kids involved. Things like, after being put in time out, Nick "refused" to stay facing the wall for the entire five minutes or for speaking out in class. I kept reminding them that they were talking about a seven year old boy. The final straw was when I was called because Nick had picked up a small stick and thrown it.

When I arrived at the school, I was told that during recess, Nick had approached two or three groups of kids looking for someone to play with. After being turned away by each group, he turned around and walked over to a tree. The playground aide said Nick sat down by the tree and, after playing in the dirt for a brief period of time, he picked up a small stick and tossed it down by his feet. At that point, he was removed from the playground and placed in Step 4.

I asked whether there were any other kids in his vicinity – and was told no. I asked if he had made any overt actions toward where the other kids were playing – and was told no. I asked if anyone was hurt by his actions – and was told no; which led me to ask why he had been removed from the playground. The principal explained that to pick up anything from the ground and throw it was a violation of the school rules and any student breaking a school rule would immediately be placed in Step 4.

I told the principal that I felt they should be less concerned about a small stick and more concerned about why one little boy was unable to find even one other child, out of the 90 or so kids on the playground, to play with. Thus, leaving the little boy feeling like it was necessary to isolate himself and sit sadly under a tree.

Without responding, the principal changed the topic and asked if anyone had ever mentioned that Nick might have ADHD. She said that Nick had trouble staying in his seat in class. She said he would often blurt out the answer when the teacher asked a question, he would turn around when someone entered the class and he liked tapping on his desk with his pencil. All of these behaviors were distracting in the classroom.

I attempted to explain how the students in his class in Missouri were encouraged to be curious about their environment and how they had been allowed to speak out when they had the answer. She asked how many children there had been in his class in Missouri. I told her I believed there were 15-18 students, with one teacher and often an aide. She told me that in the classes at this school, most teachers had 28-30 students, and sometimes more. She said the type of behavior Nick was exhibiting was unacceptable because it was distracting to the rest of the students. She suggested that I consult a psychologist and have Nick placed on medications to control his behavior. I told them that I refused to medicate my child because he acted like a child. Without waiting for a response, Nick and I left the principal's office. I have no idea whether she said anything to Nick's teacher, but the last week of school was uneventful.

In June, I started a full-time job with a nurse-staffing agency. I had heard about the Boys & Girls Club and signed both boys up for summer care. Next to the Boys & Girls Club was a school with an art based academic program. They offered classes that fostered each student's creativity. I decided to enroll all three of my children for the next school year. I would drop the kids off at the school on my way to work and they would go directly to the Boys & Girls Club when school was out, and I could pick them up after I got off work.

Nick was in a combined class of first and second graders and his brother was in a combined class of second and third graders. The first couple of months, of second grade, went by with little disruption. During the first parent-teacher conference, Nick's teacher mentioned that she had read in Nick's records that his preschool teacher suspected he might have ADHD. She asked if I had ever had him evaluated. I told her if you considered a fifteen-minute interview, when he was five years old, then being handed a prescription an evaluation – then yes, one had been done. I also told her that I had contacted his kindergarten and first grade teachers back in Missouri and both had assured me that Nick was just a normal, active little boy.

The teacher told me that Nick had trouble completing paperwork. She said he would often sit at his desk and just stare or doodle on the paper. One trait, which was particularly odd to her, occurred when she was giving the weekly spelling test. She said that she would say the word, use it in a sentence and then say it again before moving on to the next word. Often, she would be on the third or fourth word before Nick had written anything down and then suddenly, he would write the next word and go back to word one and fill in each of the missing spaces. She told me she had never seen a child do work like that. For several more minutes, she pointed out all the things that she thought were "wrong" with Nick. All the things that she thought meant he had ADHD or some other learning disability.

When she was done, I asked her if there was anything that Nick did right. She paused and then said that anytime she or one of the aids would read a story and then ask questions, Nick's hand would be the first one in the air and most times, he had the answer right. But, she was quick to add that nearly all assignments involved written work.

At that time, I had never heard of the theory of multiple intelligences (which refers to the individual way(s) each person learns), sometimes called learning styles.

Chapter 3

To Drug or Not To Drug

About mid-year, when the kids returned from Christmas break, the principal, Mrs. D. asked if Nick had been evaluated yet. I said, "No, it was my understanding that if the school wanted a child to be evaluated, they would order the testing through the school district." She was clearly upset and told me that as his parent, I should have initiated the evaluation. Clearly, I misunderstood the process involved. I felt like a failure to my son at that point.

There was no way I could take the constant calls at work, the sad expressions, and the failing grades. I caved. I told Ms. D. she could order the testing for Nick. Within 30 days, Nick had been "evaluated", and the diagnosis of ADHD was again given. I was referred to the county psychiatric services and was told they would issue the prescription and monitor his progress. So, there we were. My 8-year-old son was officially on drugs. Two little pills a day, one in the morning, before he left for school, and one at lunch. Back and forth we went to that psychiatrist's office, every other month, walk in – Hi, how are you? – Fine – And you? – Fine – Nick, how are you? – Fine – OK, step on the scale – OK – weight's fine – here are your scripts – see you in another 2 months. That was it.

Why do schools sponsor the Drug Abuse Resistance Education (DARE) program and then turn around and pressure parents to put their kids on the same class of controlled substances this program preaches kids to stay away from?

Along with the prescriptions came an Individualized Education Plan (IEP) at school. An IEP is supposed to outline the student's learning strengths and weaknesses; at least that is what I was told. Once these are identified, a plan is set out that is supposed to help the child improve their weak areas and take advantage of their strong areas. It actually was several years later that I found out that the "strengths" were supposed to be based on how a child learns, not on their personality as they were in Nick's case. I guess these plans work for some children, but for my son, nothing changed. Nick was failing at school. If anything, he was becoming more withdrawn. Nick never argued or complained. But he did change. The happy little boy that wanted to please everyone turned sullen and quiet. He tossed and turned at night, and he was hard to get up in the morning.

The school year moved on, and Nick continued to slide deeper and deeper down. One day, as I was picking the boys up, he seemed particularly sad. I asked what had happened and Nick said he heard his teacher say she hated second graders. He said that meant she hated him! I tried to make him feel better, telling him it was possible he heard it wrong or maybe he missed part of the conversation. Through his tears, he said he was right there and he heard what she said, and he knew what that meant.

The next day, I stopped in to see the principal when I dropped the kids off for school. I told her what Nick had relayed. Her initial response was, "teachers don't have favorites." After controlling a laugh, I told her that unless a robot was teaching my son, I knew firsthand that teachers had their favorites because I had been one. Along with their favorites, they also had their least favorites – just like anyone else. Together we walked over to the classroom where I relayed what Nick had told me. Instead of understanding that I was talking about the feelings of a little boy, she actually got defensive. She told me that Nick had no business listening in on an adult conversation. I reminded her that Nick was an 8 year old little boy and she, as an adult, had no right making comments like that within the hearing distance of any child. On the way back to the office, I told the principal I had my concerns about Nick continuing to be in that classroom. There was no changing his mind. He would continue to believe that the teacher hated him. She said because they used combined classrooms, the room he was in was the only one available until he passed the 2nd grade.

By the end of 2nd grade, Nick was in danger of failing. He was still convinced that his teacher hated him. For the most part, he just refused to do any written work. He continued to excel in the verbal portions of class and according to his IEP; he was to receive testing verbally.

At the end of the year, when I asked about his test scores, I learned he had been tested like all the other kids. I asked why the accommodation for verbal testing never happened and was told the shortage of teachers and aides made it impossible. I failed to understand the purpose of setting up an IEP if the school was unable to meet the student's learning needs. During the last conference, I sat with Nick's teacher and the principal.

As I reviewed Nick's work, I commented that there were some areas that he did extremely well. I asked for an assurance that he would be put in the 2nd/3rd grade combined classroom and that way he would be able to do some 3rd grade work in the subjects he was excelling in and some 2nd grade work in the subjects he was having trouble with. "Yes," the principal said, "I'm sure that can be worked out."

Summer was uneventful and because no one had explained the "addictive" nature of the medications he was on, I saw no reason to give them to him when he when school was out. The first week of August we returned to the "Welcome Back" Open House. It was the night to meet the boy's new teachers for the soon to start school year. The boys and I walked into the room that David's teacher from the year before occupied. David gave her a big hug and told her we were here so Nick could meet her because he was going to have her for his teacher. The teacher bent down and told David that his brother was in the other classroom. Perplexed, I said I was confused as this was the only 2nd/3rd grade classroom, and I had been assured at the conference, at the end of last year, that this was the classroom Nick would be this year. She told me I better talk with the principal.

I found Ms. D. in the gymnasium of the Boys and Girls Club. I asked why Nick was back in the 1st/2nd grade classroom when she had assured me, at the end of the last school year, that he would be in the 2nd/3rd grade classroom. She said Nick needed to be held back and would be in the same classroom that he had been in last year. I reminded her that Nick was unsuccessful last year partly due to his belief that the teacher hated him. I asked how she could place a boy who was going to be 9 years old in a couple of months in a class with 6 and 7 year olds. It was my understanding that she had no authority to hold my son back without my permission and I refused to give it. I told her I would never allow Nick to return to that classroom. She said, "My decision stands." I said, "Then none of my children will be attending your school."

So that was that. School was scheduled to start in less than one week and my sons had nowhere to go. I called my friend, Gina, and told her what happened. I was shaking with emotion. She suggested I let the boys go to school with her kids at the local charter school. I told her I needed someplace they could stay after school, and she said the school would bus the kids to the Boys & Girls Club, so there was no need to worry. She said their open house was tomorrow night and I could go with them.

The next night, Gina introduced me to the principal of the charter school. I explained how they had tried to put Nick in with the little kids, back in the classroom with the teacher that he felt hated him. When I told her what the principal had said about teachers not having "favorites," she chuckled and asked if they were super-human. I knew I liked this lady – she was real. She said she would put Nick in with the other kids his age, in the 3rd grade, and we would see how he did. We had returned to the psychiatrist's office and Nick was on a new regimen of pills – morning, noon and possibly in the afternoon if there were problems in his after school care. With IEP in hand, Nick started the 3rd grade in Ms. B's class. Ms. B was the best teacher. She called to see if there was a problem; she encouraged Nick to try new things. She helped him complete his daily work by reading things to him. She used to say how much Nick liked being read to. But as the months passed, Nick talked less, laughed less and seldom had a smile on his face – except for when he was with Ms. B. But even Ms. B could tell something was wrong. She finally called one day and asked if his medications had been changed. She said she thought the new meds might be too strong. She said that Nick would often sit like a zombie until around mid-morning and then all the sudden he would appear to become overly anxious almost to the point of being hyperactive. After lunch when he was sent to the nurse's office and was given the next pill, he would appear to zone out again. She said it was becoming more and more difficult to get any work out of him – unless she was working one on one or reading to him. The adults at the Boys & Girls Club reported that about 4:00pm, he would run around the Club like a "chicken with his head cut off."

The only time Nick seemed to be in control was during his weekly karate class. They were being taught intricate blocks, punches, kicks, and routines. Nick even competed in a local karate tournament and came home with a first place trophy. I was so proud and for the first time, he appeared to be proud of himself too. It never occurred to me that this change could be because there were no medications being given on the weekends and, therefore, his head was clear when he was in karate class.

Outside of karate, life stayed the same. I tried to keep the kids on a routine. Get home, fix dinner, eat together and then relax and enjoy some quiet time. Rarely did things go as planned. I love my son, I really do, but I was going nuts. His moods were all over the place. First he was happy, then he was quiet, then he was playful, then he was angry – all in a matter of 30 to 45 minutes. If I was that confused, imagine what it must have felt like inside him.

Why were some kids diagnosed with this disorder, given the pills and suddenly they were "super student" and "perfect kid." I started wondering if there was something else to this ADD/ADHD stuff. I started looking for articles online, books in the library and information in magazines. When I asked the psychiatrist, during one of our bi-monthly visits, she said she would try changing his medication, again, and see if that would make a difference. This was another new psychiatrist – seems like he rarely saw the same one more than a couple of times. This time, she took him off Ritalin and put him on Adderall. Again, no mention was made that in order to avoid the "crash" that accompanies a person when they come down from the "high" from these medications, he needed to be taking them seven days a week.

The dosage on the Adderall was different, but he was still taking two pills per day and again, no observable difference in his ability to get his work done. In addition, he also started demonstrating some behavior quarks the last month or so and now these seemed to be getting worse. Nick suddenly developed this intense interest in fire.

He told me that there was something about the "wiggly colors" that he liked to watch. He started doing this thing where he would curl up his fingers and blow across the tips, like he was blowing out a match. He never could explain why, he said it was a "habit." He also had this "tic" on the right side of his face. His eye would appear to twitch without warning. Through research, I discovered that some of these behaviors were considered side-effects from the medications.

My job involved customer service. I would answer the phone, make phone calls, and do a type of data entry all day. Rarely would a week go by that at least one phone call from either the school or the Boys & Girls Club failed to came into my work. If my bosses knew how many calls I was receiving, they would have been upset.

Nick had now been on the medications for over a year. I kept wondering when they would start working.

Due to Ms. B's amazing efforts, Nick passed third grade. Summer came and went, without giving him the medications; and it was time for fourth grade. Earlier in the year, Ms. B said she thought there was a chance that she would be teaching fourth grade next year and she could keep Nick in her classroom. Unfortunately, by the end of the year, she found out she would be teaching second grade instead. Ms. B said she would talk with Nick's new teacher and fill her in on how she had applied his strengths to overcome any behavior issues. She assured me that Nick would be fine this year. I think she is the person that told me that as the kids get older, everything gets better. Maybe for some kids, not for Nick though. The fourth grade was a mirror image of third grade with the odd behaviors, tics, and zoning in and out during the day. The big difference was the absence of Ms. B. For Nick, it was a tremendous loss.

I was finding it harder and harder to keep up with work and the responsibilities of being a single mom. The stress was overwhelming but I was raised to believe that a parent – mom or dad – took care of their responsibilities, put a smile on their face, and buried everything else deep inside. No matter what kind of pain – physical, mental, emotional, or spiritual - a parent's job was to keep going.

I had a bout with a wrist disorder back in 1995 and was told at that time that I should consider looking into another type of work than what I had been doing for years. But being a secretary or doing administrative work was pretty much all I knew. I tried starting my own business, after my divorce in 1994, but the equipment kept breaking down and I had to close it in less than a year. I returned to office work. Then in

November of 2003, the pain in my wrists started all over again. It looked like the decision was being made for me. Now I had to add physical therapy to my "stuff to do list" and the problems at school with Nick just continued. There were even problems on the bus.

Why some adults like to pick on kids, especially those that seem to be unable to defend themselves is beyond my understanding. The bus driver would have Nick and two other little boys from his class sit in the very back of the bus with the bigger boys. Nick had asked if he could sit with his brother, but the bus driver refused. Similarly, the other two boys were moved from sitting by their siblings. Unfortunately, most of the school year had gone by before my older son finally told me what was going on.

I called the bus barn. The supervisor called back and assured me that type of behavior would not be tolerated. She said the bus driver would be spoken to. She also admitted that the parents of the other two boys involved had also filed complaints. I felt like it was too much of a risk. For the remainder of the school year, I took the boys to school in the morning and would have them go to the neighborhood park and wait for me to pick them up after I got off work, one of the benefits of the weather in Arizona. There is no way that plan would have worked if we still lived in SW Missouri. I guess the world has always had characters in it like this guy. You often hear about criminals that get off by playing the power card over someone more vulnerable than they are. And you expect that from a criminal – not from a teacher, bus driver, or school administrator. I was relieved to learn that this would be his last year as a driver.

There was no improvement with Nick's grades so the next time we went to the psychiatrist's office, another new psychiatrist changed the medications again. With less than a month left in the school year, the new psychiatrist said he wanted to add a new medication to Nick's regimen. He said to give Nick 20mg of Adderall XR before school, 10mg of Adderall at noon and then a new drug, Seroquel, to help him sleep at night. I remember feeling stunned at that suggestion. I struggled to even imagine how a medical doctor, a psychiatrist, expected me to, in essence, drug an 11-year-old boy 24 hours a day. That was it. I was done with drugging my child.

After leaving the psychiatrist's office, I told Nick we were going to finish out the school year with the meds he had left and that would be it. There would be no further medications. The smile on his face said it all. He finally admitted that he hated the way the meds made him feel. I asked him why he had never said anything before now. His reply broke my heart. He said, "It's ok, mom. I'll do whatever you need me to do. I will be ok." I asked him to promise me that if, in the future, anything I did or asked him to do made him feel bad, he needed to tell me right away. "I will mom," he said with a smile.

Chapter 4
No Meds – No Education

So, without the drugs, summer began and my thoughts returned to supporting my family. Massage therapy was just beginning to really take off in the valley, so I thought about studying that. I visited a couple of the massage schools but after hearing how much stress massage puts on the wrists, I knew that would be getting out of one fry pan and right into the fire. Then I found a school in Tempe, AZ that offered classes in Energy Medicine and Spiritual Studies. An avid reader all my life, I found the idea of working with the body's energy field fascinating. I had studied Reiki in Missouri and earned the title of Reiki Master. I heard it was possible to make a good living providing healing energy services.

The summer of 2004, while still working full-time at the nurse staffing agency, I started school at the Southwest Institute of Healing Arts. It was an 18-month, Associates of Occupational Studies program in Mind-Body Psychology, which would provide me with the opportunity to open my own business or work with a holistic health or naturopathic practitioner. Classes were held in the evening and over the weekend. In the course of study, I was introduced to several different holistic modalities. The one that caught my attention was hypnotherapy. My instructor talked about being able to help people release old thoughts, traumas and recreate a person's thoughts and beliefs about themselves. She said that hypnotherapy was safe for every age. After that first weekend, I was hooked. I knew what I wanted to do. I knew I could develop a hypnotherapy program that would help kids that were like my son. I knew there had to be a way to remove the labels and restore a child's self-esteem. I excitedly set into my course of studies, each class bringing more and more clarity to my path. But as we all know, life happens, especially when we were planning for something else.

The first day of the new school year, both boys were really excited. Since I had stopped giving Nick the medications, I had been researching natural options that might help him with focus and concentration. I decided to give him a multi-vitamin, Ginkgo biloba, and Lecithin. Nick was ready for the opportunity to prove he was just like any other boy, and he was able to get things done.

When the boys got home, I asked how their day went. In turn, Nick asked why people were so quick to judge kids when they never took the time to get to know them. I asked why he would ask that question. Nick said that this morning, when they went to get on the bus, the same driver that was mean to him last year was on the bus. He said the driver was training a new driver on the route. David spoke up and said the driver had never liked Nick and a couple of the younger boys. He said when they went to get on the bus, the old driver said, "This is David and he is a good kid. This is his brother, Nick, and he is nothing but trouble. They tried to get me fired last year, but I am still here. I will show you what you need to do to get him off the bus for good." I was shocked. I called the transportation office and left a message for the supervisor. The following day, I heard back from the supervisor and after relaying the information, she said the driver was only training the new driver and would be gone in about a week. I told her I needed my boys to feel safe riding the bus. I decided to give it a week. About midway through week 2, Nick got written up. The report said he got out of his assigned seat. When I asked Nick what had happened, he said the new driver refused to let him and David sit together. He said he had to sit by this big kid and when the driver was looking away the kid pushed him into the aisle. Nick said he stood up and the bus driver yelled at him. He said he tried to tell the bus driver what happened, but the driver just told him to sit down. David confirmed that Nick was telling the truth.

I told my boss that I was pulling my kids out of the school they were going to and would need to come in late or miss the next day so I could get them registered in the new school. I ended up taking the next day off work and went to the school board to find out what elementary school served the area we lived in. I went to the school and filled out enrollment papers for both boys. I wanted the boys to attend the same school.

Looking back, it probably would have served David better if I had left him at the charter school. I know he resented Nick and thought I was playing favorites. I tried to explain that I needed him to take care of his little brother when he was the only one there. When it came to other kids picking on Nick, David was right there, but when it came to one on one with each other or competing with each other for time with me, there were times it was really bad. Was it fair to David? I would like to think it was part of being a family, but he was just a boy himself. That is the downfall of being single parent. I asked my kids to take on more responsibility and treated them more like little adults instead of the two young boys and one young girl.

Once the new school received Nick's transcripts, they called me in and asked when I would be bringing in his medications. There it was, that label again, in his permanent school records. The meeting was with the school principal and Nick's new homeroom teacher. I explained that Nick had failed to respond to the medications and the possible side effects were more than I was willing to chance. The principal said, "You need to put him back on the medications. Otherwise, we may have to transfer him to an alternative school." I asked why they would consider that since he had yet to be given him a chance to succeed. The principal said, "Our teachers are unequipped to deal with a child who was not being medicated."

I could not believe my ears. "I'm not drugging my son," I said, "He is taking a multi-vitamin and specific herbs that are know to balance the behaviors associated with ADHD. I believe they will make a difference." "He was diagnosed with a disorder, and you need to give him the medicine that will keep it under control," the principal said. "No, it is my choice as a parent," I said, and walked out of the office.

The nit picking began and within three months, they had documented enough events to recommend a transfer. Nick spoke out in class. Nick spent too much time in the bathroom. Nick rocked his chair back on two legs. Nick didn't finish his paper. Nick didn't do the assignment the right way. Nick pushed another boy in line. Nick…. Nick…. Nick….and on and on. By the end of November, the school announced that Nick would be transferred to the district's alternative school because of his emotional and behavioral problems. No matter how I objected, I was told there were no other alternatives.

Nick became more and more withdrawn. Here he was, in fifth grade, being thrown in with kids who had been in trouble with the police. Nick has never been a bad kid. He was never mean or cruel, but he was often the brunt of other kids bullying. I tried to find the "bright" side.

The school principal assured me that they would work with Nick. He would get the special education he needed. He assured me that the phone calls would stop because the school provided a secure environment in the event Nick got in trouble so I would no longer have to worry about getting calls at work. I tried to explain that the last thing Nick needed was having the work made easier for him. He like to be challenged and he was perfectly capable of doing the same work as any other child in his classroom. Despite my objections, the principal picked up where he left off, like I had said nothing at all. He went on to state that instead of the twenty spelling words that the majority of fifth grade students were given each week, Nick would only be given ten. And in math, he would be in the Special Education class so the work would be easier.

Nick spoke up at that point and said, "If you don't think I can do it, why should I bother?" The principal just kept talking. I interrupted him and asked if he heard what Nick had said. "No," he responded. I reminded him that Nick was sitting in the room with us and could understand everything he was saying. I then asked Nick to repeat what he had said. So again, Nick asked him, "If you don't think I can do it, why should I bother?"

So, this was it – this was the principal's chance to make a real difference in my son's opinion of the school environment, and his ability to learn. I was just repeating in my mind, 'Teaching moment, teaching moment,' just hoping he would take advantage of this opportunity. Instead, the principal said, "Because the law requires you to be in school until you are sixteen years of age." Phewwww.... Just like a missile crashing to Earth, Nick shut down. Unless it had relevance to his everyday life, Nick saw no point in putting any effort into schoolwork.

I told the principal that there would be no medications for my son. I would be providing herbal supplements for him to take. I had to complete paperwork advising the school nurse when to provide these supplements to Nick. Two days later, I received a call from the nurse advising that she would be unable to give Nick any 'medications' without a doctor's signature. I explained that I was giving Nick herbal supplements in place of pharmaceutical medications. The products were sold over the counter without any kind of doctor's approval required to purchase. She stated she would be unable to give Nick the supplements without a doctor's approval. I told her I had already checked with the school board and there were no regulations forbidding her from giving my son nutritional supplements. After a bit of a silence on the other end, the nurse said she would have to get back to me.

I felt like I had won one small battle. I just wondered why it had to be a battle in the first place. It took the nurse three days to get back to me but in the end, she confirmed what I already knew – the school could not stop me from giving my son nutritional supplements. I only had to bring in the bottles with my written instructions on when and how many of each supplement she should give him.

Nick's biggest problem that year was the lack of motivation to do any of the work – work he was perfectly capable of doing. True to his word, unless he could find relevance to the work, he refused to put any effort into completing the assignments. This was confirmed during one of my parent-teacher conference with his homeroom teacher. Ms. Q. said Nick was more than capable of doing the work and when she would explain to him how the work related to real life, he would comply. Ms. Q. showed me several examples of Nick's work, most having grades from the upper 80's to 100%. I was very impressed. She also said that no matter how bad Nick's day had been he would come in the next day with a good attitude. She said some of the other kids would pick on him, but he would never hold a grudge and would often try to befriend those same kids the next day. Nick's Special Education English/Reading teacher was another matter.

During this parent-teacher conference, while I was talking with Ms. Q., the other teacher entered the room like a bull charging after a red flag. You could feel the negative energy that followed her. I watched Nick's response as she entered the room. His face changed from a smile to a frown, he took one step back and then crossed his arms across his chest like he was trying to protect himself from a direct blow. This teacher ranted for almost 10 minutes about how Nick refused to do the work in her class. Finally, I interjected and relayed the information from his homeroom teacher. The English/Reading teacher became even more defensive and said, "I refuse to accept any responsibility for Nick's refusal or inability to do his work." At that, she left the room. Ms. Q and I exchanged a look, and I asked how a person with that kind of attitude could be allowed to interact with children that needed support, instead of negativity. She said it is the shortage of qualified teachers. Having a college degree should never be the only deciding factor in allowing a teacher, or any other adult, right to bully a child. Apparently, for some, being a teacher is about having power over others. Beware of any teacher that wants advance notice before you visit their classroom.

In the first decade of the 21st century, education – or least education in Arizona – was focused on teaching every child to do their work the same as every other child so they could all score high on the standardized tests. These test scores are directly linked to the amount of Federal funding the school received.

The Special Education Math teacher wanted Nick to do his math a certain way. The problem was, Nick could come up with the correct answers, but for some reason he was unable to write down all the steps he had taken to get the answer. Because of this, the problems were marked wrong. Nick did not understand. He got the right answer, but the problem was marked wrong. Frankly, it puzzled me too. When I spoke with his math teacher, he said that the math they are teaching was less about getting the right answers, and more about understanding the process to get to the answer. Nick had to learn the process to get to the answer the way it was being taught. I asked why a correct answer was being marked wrong. Again, he said it was about the process instead of about getting the right answer. That made absolutely no sense to me. I told the math teacher that I knew from experience that if my boss asked me for the answer to a problem, all he cared about was whether I gave him the right answer. The last thing he is going to care about is how I got to that answer. I asked him if the purpose of the public school system is to prepare a child to be ready for a career, maybe they should focus on enhancing the strengths of each child – even if that meant them doing the problem differently.

The continuing phone calls from school were taking their toll. In November of 2004, I was called into the office and told that my productivity had dropped off, and I was going to be written up. I reminded my boss that I had been a loyal employee since June of 2001. I had worked the office by myself, from open to close, and often worked on-call nights and weekends when there was no one else. I had taken on any additional duties, including back up payroll person, new employee trainer and out of office sales. I was attending school full-time, often working all week, and going to school two or three nights and/or all weekend. I had made the mistake of thinking that my boss was also my friend. She told me I needed to either bring up my productivity or I would be let go. Then she looked at me and said, "I really don't want to have to fire you Mary. I know how hard you have worked and I know the problems with Nick haven't helped, but I'm being pressured from Tucson" (which was where her boss's office was located). Susan said, "I have no choice. I have to put you on 30-day notice. If your numbers don't increase by the end of December, I have to let you go."

Really??? You are going to let me go right after the holidays? Well, December came and went, and two people had quit in the Phoenix office. Now the company was short a Client Services Specialist and a Payroll Specialist. So, guess who was doing the weekly payroll? Susan said, "We have decided to extend your thirty day notice until the end of January because of the vacation time you took in December (no mention of taking on all the other roles)." She said, "I have to have a full thirty days to properly evaluate your production levels." I asked if it had anything to do with the other two employees who had quit, and Susan only smiled.

January came and I was asked to train two new employees. Turns out, one was meant to be my replacement. By the second week of February, both employees were trained and I was again called into the office. I was told that my productivity had remained below an acceptable level. I asked how I was supposed to maintain my productivity, train new employees, and conduct out of office sales at the same time. I was told those activities were all considered part of my job responsibilities. Then Susan turned on the friend face and voice. She said, "I really don't want to fire you, Mary. I have held Tucson off as long as I can. They wanted me to fire you last month, but I knew you were going to graduate from the hypnosis program and I wanted to hold off as long as I could." I said I would have an answer for her by the end of the week. On Friday, I turned in my two-week notice. My last day would be Friday, the 25th of February.

Looking back on it now, I kind of wish I had let them fire me. At least I would have been able to draw unemployment and have some sort of income coming in while I figured out what my options were. My belief, at that time, was that being fired from any job was a mark against me and my abilities. I was still so worried about what other people thought of me.

I began telling some of our nurses that I would be leaving. Much to the company's chagrin, several of the nurses advised they would be leaving with me. A couple even told me the only reason they were still working for this company was because of me. Unfortunately, I had signed a non-compete so I was unable to go to work for another nurse staffing agency within a 50 mile radius of Mesa.

On my last day, I wanted to stay at work all day so I could say goodbye to a number of employees who regularly came into the office in the afternoon to pick up their paychecks. The company had other plans. At noon, instead of going to lunch, I was told I needed to turn in my key and go home. I asked to finish out the day and was told I would be paid for the full day, but I needed to leave now so they had time to change the locks.

I had completed the primary specialty, the hypnotherapy part of my program, but still had another year to complete the entire AOS Mind-Body Psychology degree. Becoming certified as a hypnotherapist meant a lot to me. I started working with Nick, working to improve his self-esteem, and convince him that he was as smart and capable as I knew in my heart he was.

I also began seeing clients. I knew I was on the right path. I began searching for information that would explain why Nick was having so much difficulty at school. I had signed up for a series of teacher-training courses. I wanted to have some idea of the training that my son's teachers might be getting. In one of the classes, which were actually geared toward post-high school teachers, information was presented

on the Theory of Multiple Intelligences, by Howard
Gardner. The theory was based on his research, at the
Harvard Graduate School of Education, in which he
identified nine different learning styles, or ways of
understanding. That really struck a nerve with me. I
recalled that at least one of Nick's teachers commented
about his strong ability to listen to information in class
and then answer questions or recite the information
back.

My next stop was the public library. I checked out
several books on learning styles and/or multiple
intelligences by several authors, including Dr. Gardner
and Thomas Armstrong, another advocate of teaching
children based on how they learn. One of the books
outlined how to teach each subject based on the child's
learning style. I was fascinated and wondered why the
public school system had failed to incorporate this into
each classroom. I was surprised to learn that this book
was written in 1924. The author, Rudolf Steiner,
founder of the Waldorf Education System, was from
Germany and this type of teaching was common in
European countries. I read other books that provided
questionnaires that helped me identify Nick's learning
style. He is a Verbal-Linguistic and Bodily-Kinesthetic
learner. What that means is that he needs to either hear

what you want from him, or he needs to literally touch - get his hands on and into - the parts involved in a problem before he can arrive at an answer. This research led me to an understanding that the reason Nick struggled in the public school system in Arizona is because they teach all students in the Logical-Mathematical learning style. Nick's brain and I was sure many other children's brains were unable to process information that way.

Do you know how your child learns? Do you know how you learn? There are a number of FREE online resources that will aid you in identifying your, or your child's, learning style. This is an awesome opportunity to identify the similarities you share with your child or children, but even more so, it gives you a chance to celebrate your differences. For me, it really helped me understand why my son responded to requests I made the way he did. It helped keep me from getting frustrated when his response was different than what I expected it to be. Now that I knew a little bit more about how his brain processed requests, I could change the way I was asking, and life would be easier for the both of us.

Armed with the information I had discovered in my research, I went to Nick's school and spoke to the principal. I asked if there was anyway Nick's assignments could be modified to fit his learning styles. The principal advised that the district dictates the way lessons are taught. Nick would just have to adjust, like every other child, and learn to do things the way the teacher was teaching them. As the school year came to a close, the administration advised that Nick had not progressed enough to go back to "regular" school and, therefore, would be attending their school again next year. I had no idea what I was going to do, but I knew that Nick would never return to that school.

My options were seriously limited. If I kept Nick from going back to the "alternative" school and the school district refused to let him go to "regular" school, then the only thing left was home schooling. Could I do that? Did I really have the skills needed to teach my son?

I felt like I had no choice, so I began checking into the multitude of homeschooling programs. Why are so many home school programs based in religion? I decided a long time ago that I would let my children choose what religious belief systems they wanted to explore, and school was no place to force beliefs on them that I was unable to even say I agreed with.

After several days of searching for information on the internet, I came across a school called Arizona Virtual Academy (AZVA). It just so happened that there was an AZVA presentation coming up at the end of the week. I found out that AZVA is a state accredited charter school that provides lesson plans, schoolbooks, and a computer system and even pays for half the cost of the internet connection. This appeared to be the answer I was looking for. I would have the support of a regular classroom teacher and a special education teacher, because of Nick's IEP, on a bi-weekly basis. I was also told if I had any questions, I could call or e-mail the teacher anytime. This assurance boosted my belief and self-confidence in my ability to be Nick's teacher. I had done my share of teaching others in the workplace over the last 20 years, but it was a lot different when it came to instructing my own child. But I knew I had to give it a shot.

Over the next two years, Nick excelled in the AZVA program. No drugs, no treating him different than any other sixth grader, and even though there was a Special Education teacher at our disposal, he would be doing the same assignments as every other sixth grader in the program. We took turns reading the assignments and I bought a set of manipulatives to help in math. In his seventh grade year, he even made the honor roll. This was the first time in his academic career that he achieved that honor. The major difference between home schooling and public school was the ability to work with Nick, one on one, in each of the assignments. I also added an aromatherapy blend to aid with concentration, continued the healthy diet changes, nutritional and herbal supplements. This is where I really want to help other parents.

Further on in your reading, you will find chapters on easy changes you can make – starting in the kitchen. Then I will help you explore a variety of natural therapies – both herbal, aromatherapy and flower essence formulas you can add to your child's daily routine. It took time, but I slowly realized that there was no single method that was going to allow children like Nick to excel in school.

Parents are going to have to look at their child's diet and exercise, be creative with lessons, get at least a basic understanding of learning styles and identify which styles they and their child were strongest in. Other options include nutritional supplements, aromatherapy, guided imagery, cranial sacral massage, cleansing the digestive tract of heavy metal toxins, and flower essences for emotional support. As a parent, you will have to decide whether to use pharmaceuticals, natural formulas, or a combination of both to address the symptoms of these childhood emotional, behavioral, and learning disorders.

At this point, I had graduated from the mind-body program and began seeing clients in addition to the home schooling. The most common question that my client's parents asked was if there were herbal alternatives for the drugs being prescribed for their children. Even though I was using herbs for my son, I was unsure whether I knew enough to really make educated recommendations. The only way to answer that question for my clients, and to find out more about options for my own son, was to return to school.

In July of 2006, I returned to SWIHA and enrolled in the AOS Holistic Health program, specializing in Western Herbalism. The Western Herbalism program stressed the obvious. If a person is suffering from symptoms of some type of disease or disorder, then something in the body is out of balance. Find the cause of the imbalance and you can eliminate the symptoms and restore overall health and wellness.

It is my deepest desire to find the answers that will save other parents and young people from the experiences Nick and I had gone through especially when it comes to the drugs commonly prescribed.

I originally saw this book as the end result of my research into discovering what body systems may be out of balance when the common symptoms of childhood diagnosed emotional, behavioral and/or learning disorders present themselves and the natural options available to them. That has changed. My mission is to continue seeking out new research that will provide a greater understanding into how and why these symptoms present themselves and finding opportunities to share this information. Keep a look out.

Chapter 5

Symptoms of Childhood Behavioral Disorders

For some reason, it is exceedingly difficult to find updated statistics on the number of children being medicated for childhood behavioral disorders. The was able to find statistics from 2007, 2011, 2018, and some for 2022-2023. The most complete statistics reported that 42.8% of children, aged 3-17, that had been diagnosed with at least one type of behavioral or emotional disorder and had been prescribed one or more psychotropic medication. It was broken down even further that 15.2% were between the ages of three and five where 50.9% were between the ages of 12 and 17.

As of 2023, of the more than seventy-three million children in the United States, 35% are between the ages of 12 and 17. Of these adolescents, 20.3% carry around a label of one or more mental, emotional or behavioral disorder. More than 60% of these diagnosed youth reported being bullied in school compared to 27.2% of non-diagnosed/labeled youths. This breaks down to an estimated 1 in 5, having a current diagnosis (HRSA, 2024). The primary treatment for these disorders is the prescribing of at least one psychotropic medication. Over one million are under the age of five (Citizens Commission on Human Rights International (CCHR), 2014). There are a number of behavioral disorders that present with mental and emotional symptoms.

The number one diagnosed childhood disorder is **Attention Deficit or Attention Deficit Hyperactivity Disorder**. This disorder is defined as a "neurobiological disorder that manifests as a persistent pattern of inattention and/or hyperactivity-impulsivity that is more frequent and severe than typically observed in individuals at a comparable level of development." Exactly what is "typically observed" anyway? Aren't observations subjective and often bias based on the person doing the observing? If you are a mom with more than one child, you typically view the behavior of your five year old little boy as it compares to your other children or your friend's children. For someone who has never had children, how can they make those assumptions? The more detailed criterion for diagnosing this disorder includes:

1. Ignores details
2. Makes careless mistakes

3. Seems to struggle with listening or following instructions
4. Fails to complete assignments
5. Loses things
6. Is easily distracted or creates distractions
7. Fidgets and squirms
8. Talks excessively, blurts out answers, or makes distracting noises
9. Has trouble waiting his turn or staying in his seat
10. Often taps fingers, feet or pencil or draws/doodles on papers

In comparison, an even more frightening discovery was the criterion used by The National Association for Gifted Children (NAGC), in Warwick, RI, to help parents and educators identify "potentially gifted" children:
1. Has high sensitivity – expresses emotions easily
2. Has excessive amounts of energy
3. Bores easily – may appear to have short attention span
4. Resists authority if it is not democratically oriented

5. Becomes easily frustrated

6. Has preferred ways of learning; particularly in reading and math – often resists rote memory or just sitting back and listening

7. Cannot sit still unless absorbed in something of their own interest

8. Is very compassionate – may fear the death or loss of loved ones

9. May give up and develop permanent learning blocks if they experience failure early

The association's website (www.nagc.org), lists a number of creative traits exhibited by these children and how these traits often surface as a problem in a traditional classroom setting. These traits include:

1. *Creative Trait:* **Theoretical and abstract** *Classroom Problem:* Ignores stressed data in assignments. Hands in "unneat" work.

2. *Creative Trait:* **Independent, Inventive** *Classroom Problem:* Resists teacher chosen assignments far beyond requirements to the exclusion of others.

3. *Creative Trait:* **Sensitive** *Classroom Problem:* Withdraws because of strong

goal orientation, peer group criticism, and rejection.

4. *Creative Trait:* **Alert, Eager**
Classroom Problem: Resents periods of classroom inactivity.

5. *Creative Trait:* **Intuitive**
Classroom Problem: Seeing conclusions without displaying knowledge of sequential concepts.

6. *Creative Trait:* **Daydreaming (as concentrated periods of thinking)**
Classroom Problem: Inattentive to teachers or classmates' comments and class discussions.

The NFGC, which was formed over 30 years ago, also stated that many gifted children tend to withdraw and may even sacrifice their creativity in an attempt to "fit in." Do you notice any alarming "coincidences" between the characteristics of ADD/ADHD and those of gifted/exceptional children?

As parents I am sure we would all prefer our children to be in the gifted/exceptional class but realistically that is impossible. Just the opposite seems to be true in the public school system. Many school administrators and teachers seem ready to jump on the ADD/ADHD bandwagon and insist parents medicate their children. How do you know which category your child fits into? Remember, the diagnosis is made based on observation only.

Begin by noting what is going on when your child acts out. If possible, spend a random day or two in your child's classroom without giving the school or teacher advance notice. Is there a specific time of day or daily occurrence (following lunch) that might be influencing the way your child acts?

In the last few years, there has been an increase in the diagnosis of **Bi-Polar Disorder** in children. This disorder is defined as a psychiatric condition with recurrent episodes of significant disturbance in mood. These disturbances can occur on a spectrum that ranges from debilitating depression to unbridled mania. Individuals suffering from bipolar disorder typically experience fluid states of mania (overly excited), hypomania (withdrawn or aloof) or what is referred to as a mixed state in conjunction with depressive episodes. In common terms, Bi-Polar Disorder is identified by extreme or not so extreme mood swings. The preceding definition currently only applies to adults because clinicians have yet to agree on the primary criteria to use to identify mania in pre-adolescent children.

If there are no recognized or widely accepted criteria for diagnosing this disorder in children, why does the number of children diagnosed with this disorder continue to rise? When did it become wrong to express your feelings openly? Happiness and sadness are often experienced in conjunction with each other. For instance, the little boy was very happy when he found a box of crayons he could color with. The little boy got very sad when his big brother took way the crayons. Is this little boy bi-polar? Maybe or maybe not – remember, there is no medical criteria for diagnosing this disorder in children.

Another thing to consider is at what age this disorder commonly appears. Remember when you started puberty? How moody were you? When young girls enter puberty and begin their menstrual cycles, it is expected that they will experience the symptoms of pre-menstrual syndrome (PMS). PMS is defined as a varied group of physical and psychological symptoms, including abdominal bloating, breast tenderness, headache, fatigue, irritability, anxiety, and depression that occur from two to seven days before the onset of menstruation and cease shortly after menses begins. However, when young boys enter puberty and they experience the same high and low spikes in their hormonal balance, they are called bi-polar or diagnosed with another type of disorder. Obviously, boys do not have menses, but they can and often do experience fatigue, headache, irritability, anxiety, and depression. I believe these behaviors should be considered normal for them.

Puberty seems to be starting earlier and earlier in kids. Could that be due to the increased use of hormone supplements in the animals that are to become the food that we eat and the food that we feed our children? Are kids being diagnosed with this disorder because of the hormonal changes occurring in their bodies? This may be one explanation why boys are more commonly diagnosed with behavioral disorders than girls. Since children spend the majority of their waking hours at school, this is where most of these behaviors are likely to show up.

Conduct Disorder is commonly diagnosed in boys who are exhibiting a pattern of repetitive behavior where the rights of others or social norms are violated. The criterion for diagnosing this disorder includes:

- Aggression
- Destruction of Property
- Deceitfulness
- Violating rules of society

Some boys are diagnosed with Conduct Disorder because they are not completing their class work or turning in their homework. This particular behavior fails to fit into the accepted criteria for this disorder, yet the disorder is often listed on school transcripts, Individual Education Plans (IEP) or 504 Plans and can affect how a child is received in future educational environments.

Before adding another label and possibly another pharmaceutical drug to your child's daily life, consider this. Children and young adults often have not figured out how to communicate their needs in a positive manner. I am not making excuses for these types of behavior; I am only offering an opportunity to explore the cause behind the behavior instead of just looking at the effect – the behavior itself.

There are blanket terms that are used to cover several different forms of abnormal, pathological anxiety, fears, phobias and nervous conditions. I've included an explanation of each here:

Anxiety Disorders are described as an irrational or illogical worry that is not based on fact. The criteria for diagnosing an anxiety disorder are dependent on the type of disorder but may include:

1. **Panic Disorder** - A psychiatric condition characterized by reoccurring panic attacks in combination with significant behavioral changes or at least a month of ongoing worry about the implications or concern about having other attacks.

2. **Post Traumatic Stress Disorder** -The term for a severe and ongoing emotional reaction to an extreme psychological trauma.

3. **Obsessive-Compulsive Disorder** - A psychiatric disorder most commonly characterized by a subject's obsessive, distressing, intrusive thoughts and related compulsions which attempt to neutralize the obsessions.

4. **Phobias** - An irrational, persistent fear of certain situations, objects, activities, or persons. The main symptom of this disorder is the excessive, unreasonable desire to avoid the feared subject.

5. **Acute Stress Disorder** - A psychological condition arising in response to a terrifying event.

According to the National Institute of Mental Health (NIMH) anxiety disorders affect about 40 million adults over the age of 18. Children can experience the same type of symptoms as adults with any of the above anxiety disorders, however, the way they react or display the symptoms if often vastly different.

How can you tell if you child has an anxiety disorder or is just going "through a phase?" Some questions you might ask include:

Does my child have an ongoing and very noticeable fear in social situations and around unfamiliar people?

Does my child experience shortness of breath or a racing heartbeat for no apparent reason?

Does my child often appear anxious when interacting with peers – or try to avoid them?

Does my child have frequent nightmares?

Does my child redo projects or papers because it was not good enough the first time?

Does my child have a persistent and exaggerated fear of an object or situation – like heights, flying or animals?

Does my child worry excessively about their competence or ability to perform?

Does my child develop physical symptoms– like stomachaches or headaches - when it is time to go somewhere they do not want to go?

Stressful events such as starting school, moving, or the loss of a parent can trigger the onset of an anxiety disorder. Some anxiety disorders tend to show up at specific stages of development. Separation anxiety disorder and specific phobias are more common in children about 6 to 9 years old.

Generalized Anxiety Disorder (GAD) and **Social Anxiety Disorder** (SAD) are more common in middle childhood and adolescence. Symptoms of GAD include:

- ☐ Restlessness
- ☐ Inability to sleep
- ☐ Fatigue
- ☐ Irritability
- ☐ Difficulty concentrating

Any of these symptoms can be triggered by normal everyday activities, such as:

- ☐ Grades/Exams
- ☐ Sports performance
- ☐ Family issues
- ☐ Health problems
- ☐ Severe weather/earthquakes

Social Anxiety Disorder is defined as extreme anxiety or fear of being judged by others or a behavior that might cause embarrassment or ridicule. This behavior may lead to withdrawal or social avoidance. Stressful events do not always have to develop into an anxiety disorder.

Encourage your child to talk to you when something is going on that they find disturbing. Sit down with your child, eye to eye, and listen to what they are telling you. Repeat back specific statements that you feel are exceptionally important for you to understand, that way the child knows that you were truly listening to what they are saying. Never underestimate the importance of any situation your child is telling you about. If you do, your child will feel that what they say means nothing to you and they will stop communicating with you.

Depression is a mood disorder that is known to have more than one cause. Psychological, biological, and environmental factors are all thought to contribute to its development. According to recent population studies, women are 1.5 to 3 times more likely to suffer from a major depressive disorder than men. It is hypothesized that the consistent rise and fall of female hormone levels may be the primary culprit. Depression is defined as a state of intense sadness, melancholia or despair that may advance to the point of being disruptive to an individual's social functioning and/or activities of daily living. No specific studies have been done and as a result, diagnosing depression in children is difficult at best. Symptoms and behaviors associated with depression in children include:

- ☐ Crying, feeling sad, helpless, or hopeless
- ☐ Feeling discouraged or worthless
- ☐ Loss of interest or pleasure in others or most activities
- ☐ Fatigue and loss of energy nearly every day
- ☐ Bad temper, irritable, easily annoyed
- ☐ Fearful, tense, anxious
- ☐ Repeated rejection by other children
- ☐ Drop in school performance
- ☐ Inability to sit still, fidgeting or pacing
- ☐ Repeated emotional outbursts, shouting or complaining
- ☐ Rarely talks to other children
- ☐ Repeated physical complaints without medical cause (headaches, stomach aches, aching arm or legs)
- ☐ Significant increase or decrease in appetite
- ☐ Change in sleep habits

Do you notice the similarities and repetition of both symptom and behavioral patterns as compared to some of the other psychological disorders already covered? At what point do we stop labeling and start looking for the cause of these behaviors?

When a child has been diagnosed with a behavioral disorder, what generally follows is an evaluation for a **learning disability.**

Learning disabilities are a group of disorders that affect a broad range of academic and functional skills including the ability to speak, listen, read, write, spell, reason and organize information which may cause the individual to have difficulty achieving at his or her intellectual level because of a deficit in one or more of the ways the brain processes information. The following learning disorders are defined and diagnosed using the following criteria:

- ☐ **Dyslexia** - Unusual difficulty sounding out letters and confusing words that sound similar
- ☐ **Dysgraphia** - Difficulty expressing thoughts on paper and with the act of writing itself characterized by problems gripping a pencil and unreadable penmanship
- ☐ **Dyscalculia** - Incomprehension of simple mathematical functions where a child often will

not perceive shapes and will confuse arithmetic symbols

- ☐ **Dyspraxia** - Difficulty performing complex movements, including muscle motions needed for talking
- ☐ **Auditory Discrimination** – Trouble distinguishing similar sounds or confusing the sequence of heard or spoken sounds
- ☐ **Dysnomia**- The inability to recall the names or words for common objects
- ☐ **Visual Perception** - The inability to differentiate between foreground and background, as well as similar looking numbers, letters, shapes, objects, and symbols
- ☐ **Attention Deficit Disorder** – Easily distracted and therefore unable to complete assignments.

When these symptoms present themselves in the classroom, the next step is an evaluation to identify what type(s) of service(s) will most benefit the child. One of the most important parts of the special education process is creating a plan for your child's education. This plan is called the Individualized Education Program, or the IEP.

The IEP is the foundation for your child's education, and you are an integral member of the team that develops it. Your child's IEP lists the specific special education services your child will receive, based upon his or her individual needs. This is why it is so important that you understand and are actively involved in developing your child's IEP. After the final IEP is established, re-read the evaluation and the recommended services over thoroughly and contact the school's psychologist if you have any questions or you disagree in any way with the information in the report.

You are the advocate for your child. Remember that this IEP will follow your child from grade to grade and from school to school. The new school administrators or teachers may never know your child on a personal level. They may be making assumptions on your child's abilities and behaviors based on the information in the transcript and file they receive. Stay on top of this. It is up to you to ensure your child is receiving the services they need. No one else will do it for you.

When children feel like their life is out of control and they have no say in their everyday activities, the one thing that they can control is what they choose to put in their mouth or fail to in some cases. The result is often an **Eating Disorder**.

An eating disorder is a complex compulsion to eat in a certain way, which disturbs physical, emotional, and psychological health. Some symptoms of various eating disorders are:

Symptoms of **Anorexia nervosa** include:

- ☐ Decreased appetite
- ☐ Poor self-esteem
- ☐ Fear of gaining weight
- ☐ Inability to eat
- ☐ Extreme weight loss

Symptoms of **Bulimia nervosa** include:

- ☐ Binge eating
- ☐ Purging
- ☐ Vomiting
- ☐ Use of laxatives or enemas
- ☐ Use of diuretics
- ☐ Fear of gaining weight
- ☐ Excessive exercise
- ☐ Poor self-esteem

As a parent, you will be the most influential factor in shaping your child's body image and eating lifestyle. Because children often take comments literally and believe what is said is factual, simple statements like – Look at that little pouchy tummy – can often leave a child feeling bad about their body. When there is conflict in the home, especially when children attempt to exert their independence, a child's eating habits are often the first to suffer. They will often overeat or even refuse to eat all together. This is a way to express their ability to control their life.

Autism Spectrum Disorders are defined as brain development disorders characterized by impairments in social interaction and communication, and restricted and repetitive behavior, all exhibited before a child is three years old. Autism can affect many parts of the brain; up until now, little to no scientific research has been conducted on the actual cause of this disorder. Because parents usually notice signs in the first two years of their child's life, there is speculation that the number of, or ingredients in, childhood vaccines may be an underlying factor. Early behavioral or cognitive intervention can help children gain self-care, social, and communication skills. The criterion for diagnosing autism spectrum disorders includes:

- ☐ Head banging
- ☐ Rocking objects
- ☐ Rocking their body

- ☐ Late speech
- ☐ Spinning objects
- ☐ Spinning themselves
- ☐ Withdrawn behavior
- ☐ Compulsive behaviors

Sometimes the syndrome is divided into low-, medium- and high-functioning autism (LFA, MFA, and HFA), based on IQ thresholds, or on how much support the individual requires in daily life. These subdivisions are not standardized and are controversial. There is an on-going debate regarding the cause of Autism. I believe that like many of the other disorders listed, the cause will never be narrowed down to just one thing.

In April 2008, the head of the CDC (Center for Disease Control) admitted that the number of immunizations given before the age of two may indeed have some bearing on a child developing Autism. In the 1950's, children received four vaccines against diphtheria, tetanus, pertussis, and smallpox. At that time, autism was virtually unheard of and affected less than 1 in 100,000 children. When I first authored this book, 1 in 68 American families had an autistic child. As of 2022, 1 in 33 children, in the United States, have been diagnosed and 1 in 5 children have been classified with some type of learning disability. All of my children received their immunizations, and I feel very blessed that they are all doing well. But just over the last ten years more immunizations have been added to the regime. I now have grandchildren, and I have told their parents that if it were me, I would require a greater spacing between the immunizations and only allow the doctor to give them one at a time. This would be purely precautionary on my part. I believe that vaccinations alone are causing the problems. My research has shown that it is the suspension agents used in the shots that contain an extremely long list of toxic ingredients, including mercury – which is any amount is considered highly toxic – even by the CDC. Why pharmaceutical companies are allowed to use toxic ingredients in these formulas is beyond my understanding.

Schizophrenia is a psychiatric diagnosis that describes a mental illness characterized by impairments in the perception or expression of. It is a severe mental disorder characterized by two kinds of symptoms; positive psychotic symptoms - thought disorder, hallucinations, delusions, and paranoia or bizarre delusions or disorganized speech and thinking in the context of significant social or occupational dysfunction - and negative symptoms – impairment in emotional range, energy, and enjoyment of activities. These symptoms must persist for at least one month and usually result in severe impairment in job and/or social functioning before a formal diagnosis is made.

The symptoms outlined for diagnosing this disorder include:

- ☐ Delusions
- ☐ Hallucinations
- ☐ Odd and eccentric behavior and/or speech
- ☐ Unusual or bizarre thoughts and ideas
- ☐ Confusing television and dreams with reality
- ☐ Confused thinking
- ☐ Extreme moodiness
- ☐ Paranoia
- ☐ Severe anxiety and fearfulness
- ☐ Difficulty relating to peers and keeping friends
- ☐ Withdrawn and increased isolation
- ☐ Decline in personal hygiene

Oppositional Defiant Disorder is a controversial psychiatric category listed in the Diagnostic and Statistical Manual of Mental Disorders (DSM -IV) where it is described as an ongoing pattern of disobedient, hostile, and defiant behavior toward authority figures that goes beyond the bounds of normal childhood behavior. The criteria for diagnosis of this disorder include:

- ☐ Negativity
- ☐ Defiance
- ☐ Disobedience
- ☐ Hostility directed toward authority figures
- ☐ Frequent temper tantrums
- ☐ Argumentativeness with adults
- ☐ Refusal to comply with adult requests or rules
- ☐ Deliberate annoyance of other people
- ☐ Blaming others for mistakes or misbehavior
- ☐ Acting touchy and easily annoyed
- ☐ Anger and resentment
- ☐ Spiteful or vindictive behavior
- ☐ Aggressiveness toward peers

All children exhibit oppositional behavior from time to time, particularly when tired, hungry, stressed or upset. Children may argue, talk back, disobey, and defy parents, teachers, and other adults, often as a means of expressing their independence. Oppositional behavior is a normal part of development for two to three year olds, commonly referred to as the "terrible two's," as well as early adolescence, or puberty. However, when a child's openly uncooperative and hostile behavior becomes a sincere concern or when it is so frequent and consistent that it stands out when compared with other children of the same age and developmental level and when it affects the child's social, family, and academic life, there may be more than normal defiance involved. However, in children with **Oppositional Defiant Disorder (ODD),** there is an ongoing pattern of uncooperative, defiant, and hostile behavior toward authority figures that seriously interferes with the child's day-to-day functioning.

The debate continues as to why the number of children being diagnosed with these disorders is rising. Is it because the symptoms for each of these disorders are becoming more defined – or in some cases more broad and overlapping? Or is it because it is easier to put a label on a behavior you dislike and then prescribe a medication to treat the symptoms instead of finding out where the original cause of the behavior began?

Of the above listed disorders, Attention Deficit Disorder (ADD) and Attention Deficit Hyperactivity Disorder (ADHD) are the most commonly diagnosed. The boom in the diagnosis began in the early 1990's. This rise in diagnosis and medications coincided with the passage of a Federal law (1991) that gave school districts an additional $400.00 for each child that is diagnosed with learning or behavioral disorder. This law was meant to buffer a major cut in educational funding that occurred at the same time. Instead, it has become a way to fund school operational budgets.

By 2003, the National Institute of Health (NIH), a division of the U.S. Department of Health and Human Services, (DHHS) estimated between 4%-6% of the **general population** suffered from Attention Deficit and Attention Deficit Hyperactivity Disorders. However, for most states, the number of children diagnosed and medicated is far above that average.

One example dates back to 1992 when the prescriptions written for psycho-stimulant medications used to treat childhood behavioral disorders in North Carolina were reported at 24,584 according to the state's Medicaid Program. In six years, by 1998, that number had increased to 135,057, which was an increase of over 550%. In the same report, the use of antidepressants in 1992 was reported at 1,326; however, by 1998 that number had risen by over 1,200% to a whopping 25,392 prescriptions.

In 2003, the Center for Disease Control conducted two statewide surveys based on the records for state sponsored medical treatment. The percentages listed in these surveys failed to list diagnosis or treatment through private medical services. The first survey compared the percentage of children aged 4-17 years ever diagnosed with ADHD by age, sex, and medication treatment status in the United States. The results ranged from 2% of 4 yr old males to 15% of 14 and 16 yr old males and approximately 0.5% of 4 yr old females and 6% of 11 and 17 yr old females have ever been diagnosed with this disorder. For those children that are taking medications, the numbers ranged from 1% of 4 yr old males to 9% of 10 and 12 yr old males and approximately 0.25% of 4 yr old females to 4% of 9, 10 and 11 yr old females. The second survey compared the percentage of children aged 4-17 years ever diagnosed with ADHD by medication treatment status and state/area in the United States. The results of this survey showed that overall, 8% of 4-17 year old children had ever been diagnosed with ADHD and 4.5% of these children were currently being medicated.

The data available on the CDC website in 2025 shows an increase in the diagnosis of these disorders by observation from 1994-2011. Remember, there are no medical tests that provide a definitive diagnosis for this disorder. In the United States, between 13% to 20% of children are diagnosed with some type of mental disorder in any given year and by 2010 it was reported that suicide, which may result from the interaction of mental disorders and other factors, including the use of pharmaceutical treatments prescribed for these disorders, was the second leading cause of death among children aged 12–17 years. The report also included data on the diagnosis rate of Attention-Deficit/Hyperactivity Disorder (6.8%) as the most prevalent parent-reported current diagnosis among children aged 3–17 years; followed by behavioral or conduct problems (3.5%); anxiety (3.0%); depression (2.1%); autism spectrum disorders (1.1%); and Tourette's Syndrome (0.2% among children aged 6–17 years). Approximately 4.7% of young people aged 12–17 years reported an illicit drug use disorder in the past year; 4.2% reported an alcohol abuse disorder in the past year; and 2.8% had cigarette dependence in the past month. For individuals under the age of 18, adverse reactions to the stimulant medications most commonly prescribed for ADD/ADHD, and requiring an emergency room visit, increased by over 4,000 between 2005 and 2010.

The most recent survey is 2011 and it shows a much larger percentage of children receiving a diagnosis of ADHD from healthcare providers than previously thought (Centers for Disease Control, n.d.).

The data and statistical information received from parental reports includes:

- The percentage of children with an ADHD diagnosis continues to increase, from 7.8% in 2003 to 9.5% in 2007 and to 11% in 2011.
- Rates of ADHD diagnosis increased an average of 3% per year from 1997 to 2006 and an average of about 5% per year from 2006 to 2011.
- Approximately 11% of children 4-17 years of age (6.4 million) have been diagnosed with ADHD as of 2011.
- Boys (13.2%) were more likely than girls (5.6%) to have ever been diagnosed with ADHD.
- The average age of an ADHD diagnosis is seven (7) years of age.
- The prevalence of an ADHD diagnosis varies state by state.

According to the National Institute of Mental Health (NIMH) page of the National Institute of Health (NIH) website, the Centers for Disease Control and Prevention's National Health and Nutrition Examination Survey (NHANES) provides the most predominance of data available is for children ages 8 to

15 which reports about 13% of these children had been diagnosed with some type of mental disorder within the last year. Of this population, it is no surprise that the most commonly diagnosed disorder is attention-deficit/hyperactivity disorder (ADHD). The data states this disorder affects 8.5% of these children. In addition, mood disorders are diagnosed at 3.7%, and major depressive disorders at 2.7% (NIMH, n.d.).

More statistics from the National Institute of Health **estimated the percentage of affected children** for the following disorders at:

Mood Disorders...............................3.7%

Conduct Disorder............................2.1%

Anxiety Disorders...........................0.7%

General Anxiety Disorder....................0.3%

Major Depression............................2.7%

Dysthymia (Neurotic Depression)............1.0%

Eating Disorders...........................0.1%

Panic Disorders............................0.4%

Autism Spectrum Disorder   1 in 68 of 8 year olds

Bi-Polar Disorder   Up to 3% of adolescents

The following statistics represent the top five states based on the percentage of youth diagnosed with

ADHD in 2023 and compares it with the statistics gathered in 2007. Most of these states have shown notable increases in **diagnosis** rates over the years:

State	2007	2023
Mississippi	7.0%	15.2%
Louisiana	11.7%	10.6%
South Carolina	9.5%	14.6%
Maine	10.0%	13.9%
West Virginia	10.0%	13.8%

Only Louisiana has shown a reduced number of children labeled with this disorder.

In comparison, the following statistics represent the top five states based on the percentage of each state's youth medicated for ADHD in 2023 and compares it with those medicated back in 2007.

State	2007	2023
Mississippi	5.8%	11.5%
Louisiana	8.3%	10.6%
Montana	3.7%	10.2%
South Carolina	6.9%	10.0%
Maine	4.6%	9.6%

These numbers are even more alarming because none of these states made it to the top ten list of states diagnosing or medicating their youth when the original statistics were collected back in 2007.

When comparing the statistics from 2007 to 2023, very few states have actually lowered the percentage of diagnosed and/or medicated children. The question must now be asked. No matter which set of statistics you look at, almost every state is diagnosing and/or medicating more children than even the American Psychiatric Association reports to have ADHD. What do these numbers tell you? What is the real purpose for the over diagnosis and medicating of our children? Before we look into that, I would like you to take a look at the diagnosis tools used by members of the psychiatric and medical communities.

Chapter 6

Diagnosing These Disorders

There are a number of diagnostic tools that can be utilized to diagnose these disorders. The preferred tool is a **Professional Psychiatric Evaluation**. This evaluation involves the use of a number of questionnaires that have been developed to assess childhood mood and behavioral disorders. They include:

- The Children's Depression Inventory (CDI), Kovacs - 1985:
- Beck Depression Inventory (BDI), Beck, Ward, Mendelson, Mock & Erbaugh - 1961:
- Reynolds Adolescent Depression Scale (RADS), Reynolds - 1986:
- Children's Depression Scale (CDS), Tisher and Lang - 1983:
- Diagnostic Interview Schedule for Children (DISC), Shaffer, and Fischer - 1998:
- Adolescent Antisocial Self-Report Behavior Checklist, Kulik et al. - 1968:

- Eyberg Child Behavior Inventory, Eyberg & Robinson - 1983:
- Family Interaction Coding Pattern, Patterson - 1982.

The advent of computer-driven assessment tools, such as the *NIMH Diagnostic Interview Schedule for Children*, Shaffer et al. - 1996, comes in a spoken version that can be given through headphones to children and/or their parents. This evaluation tool promises to greatly improve the ability of professionals outside of the mental health field to obtain diagnostic information.

Along with the professional evaluation tools, a **Parent and Teacher Evaluation** is included in the process. The instruments used by parents and teachers include the *Child Behavior Checklist,* Achenbach & Edelbrock -1983, to assess a full range of behavioral and emotional symptoms and disorders from the perspective of adult informants. The *Millon Adolescent Personality Inventory* (MAPI), Millon et al. - 1982, may be used with adolescents to assess normal and abnormal personality function.

The handbook for mental health professionals that list different categories of mental disorders and the

criteria for diagnosing them is called the **DSM-IV.**
The **Diagnostic and Statistical Manual of Mental Disorders (DSM)** is recognized worldwide by clinicians and researchers as well as insurance companies, pharmaceutical companies, and policy makers.

The **Child Conflict Index**, published in 1990 for parents of children age 2 to 12, measures problematic parent-child interactions in the home with separate girl and boy versions. The index was intended for two applications: first, to compare the outcome of a brief intervention between different families having children aged 2 to 12 years old; and second, to reflect daily variation in child behavior problems, so that other daily measures, like chronic stress, could be ascertained.

The assessment is usually conducted via telephone interview and takes approximately ten (10) minutes. Is ten minutes long enough to make a diagnosis that may affect a child for the rest of their life?

The majority of these assessments were created between 30 and 50 years ago. The newest evaluation tool was created in 1998 – over 25 years ago. Though some basic guidelines would be acceptable, it would just make sense to modify or update the criteria used to diagnose these disorders based on the modern day children? Is it really fair to today's children to be "judged" by the guidelines of a generation or two ago?

Chapter 7
Search for a Cause

Though the actual cause of these mental, emotional, and behavioral disorders is unknown and, as of this writing, there are no medical tests that can provide a physical diagnosis for the development of these disorders. Most medical and holistic practitioners commonly agree that biological imbalances may have something to do with it. Examples include:

Genetics – Did your child inherit their disorder? There is a belief from Traditional Chinese Medicine (TCM) that says that we carry our ancestor's karma seven generations – both from our past and into our future. Have you ever heard someone say, "Thoughts become things"? Think about that for a minute. If you have ever heard a relative talk about the various illnesses their ancestors had and how they were probably going to get at least one of them, isn't it possible that because of their strong belief they may have just manifested that illness by believing their relative was going to pass it on?

Chemical Imbalance – Where is the imbalance in the brain and can balance be restored? If a chemical imbalance exists, why is it there? Is it because nutritional deficiencies have failed to supply the necessary nutrients for the neurotransmitters in the brain to develop properly? Have there been other environmental influences that are disrupting the chemical composition of the brain?

Heavy Metal Toxicity – The presence of heavy metal and chemical toxins has been traced to the development of both Dementia and Alzheimer's disease in older age. The symptoms listed for both of these disorders are coincidently similar to the symptoms of many of the childhood mental, emotional and behavioral disorders. Both heavy metal and chemical toxicity accumulates in the cell neurons and increases the formation of free radicals. The heavy metal toxic substances come from mercury fillings, fish, cosmetics, pesticides, paint, plastics, fungicides, fabric softeners, contact lens solutions, soft drink cans, cookware, cheeses, baking powder, deodorant, white flour, tap water, antacids, toothpaste, laxatives, and aerosol sprays, which travel directly to the brain.

Rheumatoid Arthritis was so rare 25 years ago that statistics were unavailable and now there are over 300,000 children affected with this disorder.

The diagnosis of both **asthma** and **bowel disorders** have increased over 4 times what they were

50 years ago. There are holistic theories that provide some explanation as to the root cause of these disorders if you have that belief system. There are herbal, essential oil and flower essence therapies that may restore balance and ease the symptomatic episodes.

Questions are also arising whether the increase in **autoimmune disorders** in children are related to the heavy metal content in vaccinations or vitamin/mineral deficiencies from the food they are eating. Before a child reaches 18 months of age, they will have received up to 27 vaccinations on the 2025 schedule, sometimes as many as 6 or 7 in a single doctor's visit. Seven vaccines injected into a 13 lb. infant are equivalent to 70 doses in a 130 lb. adult. What would you say to a doctor that suggested you get 70 shots at once?

Psychological influences – which are commonly debated as to whether they are caused by Nature or Nurture. Does your child act the way he does because of a heredity factor or because of the physical or cultural environment in which he has been raised? This is not an attempt to blame the parents for their child's behavior. There are some that find that the easiest path to follow, some who choose to accept little or no responsibility for their behavior. In this case, it is merely an attempt to discover the underlying cause of the disorder or behavior pattern. What is the child getting out of the behavior? All behaviors deliver some benefit, often it is simply getting the attention they feel is lacking.

Spiritual or Environmental Influences - such as Abuse whether it be physical, mental, or emotional, because children take in everything that is said, not said, or done to them as truth. They often develop very poor self-esteem and believe themselves unworthy of achieving success in school or in life. Guided imagery combined with essential oil and/or flower essence therapy can often restore damaged self-esteem.

Stress – from peer pressure, test anxiety, the desire to be popular with teachers or peers, the desire to do well in school and the fear of failure – wondering if they are good enough – or if they will be able to please the people that are most important in their lives. Essential oil therapy is often helpful for times when you feel an anxiety or stress reaction coming on. This will be covered in a future chapter.

Relationships with family and friends – Is there an ongoing conflict or turmoil in the home or school environment?

Death of close family member or friend – For many adults, death is a concept that is hard to accept. For a child, the concept of death is difficult to understand and as a result is often associated with abandonment. Many children believe themselves to be responsible for the loss of the important person in their life. Flower Essence therapy is immensely helpful when a child or adult is under emotional stress. Again, more on that in a future chapter.

Nutritional imbalances - such as vitamin or mineral deficiency – are often caused by a poor diet, often referred to as SAD (Standard American Diet). There is an entire chapter on simple things you can do at home to help restore nutritional balance – know I would never ask you to throw everything that is yummy out of the house. Based on the Traditional Chinese Medicine (TCM) 5 Element Perspective, each element is associated with specific nutrients, organs, and behaviors. For example, an individual (of any age) who is frustrated, indecisive, angry, and/or impatient would be demonstrating an imbalance in the wood element or a liver imbalance. This can be caused by a deficiency in Vitamins A, C, K, lecithin, essential fatty acids, glutathione, or amino acids. There are both herbs and foods that are filled with these nutrients that a practitioner trained in holistic nutrition can explain this connection and help identify which nutrients your child might be missing in their diet.

Poor Nutrient Assimilation – often some type of cleanse is necessary to remove toxicities or other blockages that are preventing the proper assimilation of nutrients from the food being eaten or the supplements being taken. This area will be discussed in the chapter on nutrition.

Blood Sugar Irregularities - high and low blood sugar levels can lead to serious health issues – Type 1 Diabetes in children has increased over 17 times in children from what it was in the 1950's, from 1 in 7,100 children to 13,000 children every year in the United States. One of the Food Pyramids used in determining what foods are provided in schools has "whole grains" as a primary ingredient. Little thought is given to the fact that processed foods contain little or none of the actual "whole" grain by the time it hits the table. Also, most grains turn into sugar in the body. Do we really need more sugar in our children's diets? There is a specific herb that does an incredibly good job of balancing blood sugar. If the sugar reading is too high, it brings it down and if it is too low, it will bring it up. It is important to note that using herbal therapies does not give a person license to continue eating all the junk food on the planet.

Thyroid Deficiencies or Excesses – can affect every system within the body, including behavior, sleep, reflexes, and skin, hair, or nails. There are some theories that eating an abundance of grains/gluten or an imbalance in the beneficial bacteria in the digestive system may contribute to the apparent increase in imbalances in thyroid hormone secretion by the thyroid gland.

Adrenal Gland Depletion – caused by excessive stress. When a child experiences fear or trauma that triggers the "fight, flight or freeze" response from the sympathetic nervous system, the adrenal glands send out epinephrine or norepinephrine. This repetitive response lessens the adrenals gland ability to provide these important substances. The adrenal glands also secrete cortisol during stressful times. Too much cortisol can interfere with the pancreas' ability to produce insulin and process the sugars in our diets. There are two herbs, which will be covered later, that have a specific affinity for the adrenal glands.

Chapter 8

After the Diagnosis

You and your child have gone through one or more evaluations, and you are told your child has one or more of the above listed disorders.

Now what do you do?

Well, you can take the prescription(s) the psychiatrist gives you; go to the nearest pharmacy and start teaching your child that a little pill makes everything all better. The next chapter will go into greater detail on things you may want to consider before choosing this option.

Or you can begin a search to discover the cause of the behavior(s) your child is exhibiting.

If you choose option #2, here are some steps you can follow:

See your child's pediatrician and ask the doctor to order blood work to determine vitamin and mineral, heavy metal, blood sugar, and thyroid levels. It is important to understand that the results of blood work are based on what is going on in the body at that time, not necessarily a clear picture of what levels of vitamins and minerals your child is actually taking in. You may want to look into having a hair analysis done.

This test can actually evaluate nutritional levels back several months. You may have to make a few calls around to find someone that can perform this analysis. When the results are in, get a copy from the doctor and make an appointment to see a Naturopathic or Homeopathic Doctor, an Herbalist, Nutritionist, or other holistic healthcare provider who can explain the results of the blood work.

The practitioner you go to will probably explain how a high count of heavy metals in the blood stream, a vitamin or mineral deficiency, high or low blood sugar or a high or low thyroid hormone count may be the cause of at least some of the behavior issues. Another cause may be sensitivity to certain types of foods, including dairy products, food dyes, artificial sweeteners, wheat products, or processed food products. The food sensitivities can be determined through the use of kinesiology or delayed food allergy testing.

Applied Kinesiology is a form of diagnosis using muscle testing as a primary feedback mechanism to examine how a person's body is functioning. The doctor or health care practitioner will tell you to stick out your non-dominant arm (that means that if you are right handed, you need to stick out your left arm) and resist the pressure. You will be asked a series of questions that often require a simple one or two word answer. After you respond, the practitioner will apply a light pressure to the outstretched arm. It will feel like she is trying to push your arm down after she told you not to let her do it. With some answers, your arm will remain firm but with others, your arm will fall down like a limp biscuit no matter how hard you try to hold it up.

To put it simply, the body has within and surrounding it an electrical network or grid. Everyone has experienced that feeling when after shuffling across a carpeted floor you reach out and touch something metal or another living being and get that little shock. If anything impacts your electrical system that does not maintain or enhance your health and your body's balance; your muscles, when physical pressure is applied, are unable to hold their strength. This means, if pressure is applied to an individual's extended arm while his body's electrical system is being adversely affected, the muscles will weaken, and the arm will not be able to resist the pressure. If the body's electrical system is overloaded or has short-circuited, it causes a weakening of that system. However, if pressure is applied while his electrical system is being positively affected, the circuits remain strong and balanced and the muscles will remain strong, the person will easily resist, and the arm will hold its position.

This electrical/muscular relationship is a natural part of the human system. Kinesiology is a recognized method of reading the body's balance through the balance of the electrical system at any given moment. This method of body testing is so easy any parent can learn how to test their children for food sensitivities. A common philosophy is "the body doesn't lie." Older children can learn how to do muscle testing on themselves; and parents can teach their younger kids how to do it and make a game of it.

The simplest method to do muscle testing on yourself is by standing up straight with your feet together and your hands by your sides. Close your eyes and ask yourself a question that you know you can answer YES to – like; my name is _____? (Fill in your true name). Notice whether you feel drawn to fall forward or backward. Make a note which direction you fell toward as this is your "TRUE" direction. Next, ask yourself a question that you know the answer is "NO" to – like simply filling in the blank with a name that belongs to someone else. You should fall the opposite direction you fell in response to your "TRUE" question.

When using this method of muscle testing, you can actually hold the object in your hands and ask your body if this object is "GOOD" for you. Depending on the direction you fall, you will know whether you should be eating this food/food product – or not. Now granted, this is not a medical test to determine whether you are allergic to the food product but believe me, if you get a "NO" response and you actually stop eating whatever it was you were testing, you will feel a whole lot better. You may not be "allergic" to the product, but your body will know whether it is something that will provide the nutrition you need to succeed.

This method can be used to help children choose healthy foods at the grocery store. When your child asks you if they can have something, have them hold the product close to their body, close their eyes, and ask their body if they should have it. If they get a positive response, let them put the item in the cart. If they get a negative response, they have to return the item to the shelf and look for something else.

A second method of muscle testing is to make interlocking loops with your thumb and forefingers on both hands. Ask your YES question and then attempt to pull the finger loops apart. You should not be able to separate your finger loops if you are telling the truth. Next ask the NO question and you should be able to easily separate the loops. The difference between these two methods of muscle testing is limited to your ability to hold an item in your hands while using the finger loop method.

So now you have discovered if there are any vitamin or mineral deficiencies and whether there are any food sensitivities. The next observation is to look for reactions to your child's typical diet. Begin by keeping a five day food diary, making note of everything your child eats and drinks, along with the time of day and whether you notice any changes in your child's behavior within thirty (30) minutes to one hour after eating or drinking something.

Everywhere we turn, people are jumping on the bandwagon to change healthcare because it fails to effectively meet the needs of the people. One group, The Institute of Functional Medicine, is calling for a shift in the disease-centered focus of medical care to a patient-centered approach, addressing the needs of the whole person not just the symptoms. This is the perspective that holistic practitioners have been using for centuries.

Many medical practitioners have not been trained to explore the underlying cause of these disorders, let alone treat them on a physical, mental, emotional, and spiritual level. Holistic or alternative medicine involves understanding the origin, treatment, and prevention of further ailments. They focus on patient-centered care integrated with the newest scientific findings that combine internal and external factors that affect the ability of the body to function in a balanced manner. The time has come to change healthcare to focus on prevention, including educating the general public on nutrition, diet, and exercise.

A holistic nutrition practitioner will put together the results of all the testing and provide you with a protocol that will address:

- Lifestyle Changes – which will include exercise, relaxation, and/or work environments
- Dietary Changes – which may include the types of foods to avoid due to food sensitivity or behavioral reaction
- Herbal, Essential Oil, Flower Essence, and/or Supplementary suggestions – specifically designed to address vitamin/ mineral deficiencies or to support the specific mental /

emotional issues brought up during the initial assessment

- Dosage protocol – how much and how often your child should use these formulas or dietary supplements
- Comments – what you are doing right –
  - o Everyone needs to be told they are doing a good job!
- Products recommended – if commercial products will meet the needs of the client, or if the practitioner is unable to fill the recommended formula, options can be provided as to where you can buy the product or get the formula filled.

Depending on the results of the initial assessment and results of any medical tests recommended, the practitioner will request an initial follow up in 30 days and will ask for your and your child's input along with that of your child's teacher regarding any changes in behavior. At this point, the practitioner may change the formula or make other suggestions – or – if positive changes are being seen in the child's behavior, a continuation of the protocol will be recommended.

The duration for the use of herbal therapies is commonly one month for each year the individual has experienced the symptoms. The goal for the use of natural therapies is to return the body to the balance it was originally created with.

Chapter 9

Pharmaceutical Treatments & Side Effects

Dramatic increases have occurred over the past decade in the use of pharmacological therapies for children and adolescents with mental and behavioral disorders, but research has lagged behind the surge in their use. The gaps in knowledge span three areas in particular.

For most prescribed medications, there are no studies of safety and efficacy for children and adolescents. This is true for medications for mental disorders as well as for somatic, or body, disorders. Depending on the specific medication, evidence may be lacking for short-term, or more commonly, for long-term safety and efficacy. The problem is even more pronounced with newer medications, most of which have been introduced into the market for adults. There is often limited information about pharmacokinetics, or how a drug concentrates in body fluids and tissues over time. Most of what is known about pharmacokinetics comes from studies of adults. Pediatric pharmaco-kinetic studies are crucial to identifying the appropriate dose and dose frequency for children of different ages and body sizes.

The dosage information on over the counter (OTC) medications is written for a 150 lb. individual. Sometimes there is a child dosage protocol listed based on age. However, because not every child is the same height, weight, and body type as every other child at any particular age, parents need to know how to adjust the dosage to meet their child's specific needs. The combined effectiveness of pharmacological and multiple modality treatments are seldom studied.

The use of multiple modality treatments has the potential to yield dose reductions in pharmacological treatments, thereby improving the side-effect profile, parental acceptance, and patient compliance.

The Food & Drug Administration (FDA) has approved over 25 pharmaceuticals, both stimulant and non-stimulant, for the treatment of ADD/ADHD. The most common drug prescribed is still Ritalin (Methylphenidate HCL), also known as sustained release Concerta, Ritalin SR and Metadate CD. The FDA classifies each of these drugs as Class 2 Controlled Substance, just like Cocaine. Ritalin increases blood flow to the basal ganglia portion of the brain, which controls movement; and decreases blood flow to the frontal lobe or reasoning part of the brain, both the anterior portion which controls the "higher cognitive functions" such as planning, organizing, problem solving, behavior, attention and emotions and the posterior region which controls movement. The onset of action is relatively short at 20-30 minutes; however, the duration of the medication is often only 2-4 hours. The "withdrawal" that occurs when the drug begins to wear off may cause anxiety or agitation. No specific evidence exists to clearly establish how methylphenidate produces its mental and behavioral effects in children.

The number two most prescribed medication is Dexedrine (generic name -Dextroamphetamine Sulfate). Dexedrine is about twice as potent as Ritalin; however, because the Physician's Desk Reference (PDR) lists this medication for use as a diet control drug; it is often not covered by insurance for the treatment of ADHD. Dexedrine lasts about one hour longer, at the same dosage level, as Ritalin and the drop off is not as dramatic as that which occurs with Ritalin.

The number three drug is Adderall, which is also an amphetamine or stimulant drug. Stimulant medications have a direct action on the Central Nervous System. It is believed that Adderall's therapeutic affect may be more subtle that Ritalin and may last between 6-9 hours per dose. However, my experience with giving this drug to my son was that it only lasted about 4 hours and the crash was substantial. Adderall is most commonly used for impulse control. It is known, however, to have a distinct anorexic effect so diet management must be monitored closely in children.

Because amphetamines have a high potential for abuse, it is recommended that the medications should be discontinued periodically to determine whether the symptoms are reoccurring and if there is still a need for the medication. In most cases, however, this is never done, and some children end up taking these drugs, on a continuous basis, for up to ten years or sometimes more. For children who cannot take or who show no improvement in behavior while taking stimulant medications, anti-depressants are often prescribed. Even when anti-depressants are prescribed for ADHD, there may be no indication that the child is in any way clinically depressed. The most commonly prescribed anti-depressants for the treatment of ADHD are:

- Imipramine HCL (Tofranil, Janimine)
- Desipramin HCL (Norpramine, Pertofrane)
- Amitrtriptyline (Elavil)

- Nortriptyline (Pamelor)
- Bupropion HCL (Wellbutrin)
- Sertraline HCL (Zoloft)
- Paroxetine HCL (Paxil)
- Fluoxetine HCL (Prozac)

As of this writing, none of these medications have been approved by the FDA for use by anyone under the age of 18 and no known clinical trials have been conducted on this age group. The use of anti-anxiety medications is fairly new for the treatment of ADHD when the side effects of stimulant medications are poorly tolerated or they are ineffective.

Currently there are over 300 pharmaceuticals being prescribed for bi-polar disorder and other mental, emotional, and behavioral disorders including:

- 40 Anti-Anxiety and Sedative Drugs
- 3 Drugs for Side Effects
- 159 Antidepressants
- 72 Antipsychotics
- 77 Mood Stabilizers
- 4 to treat the Side Effects of other medications

Many of these drugs were originally designed to treat a specific disorder but are currently being prescribed to treat side effects of other prescription drugs. For example, the drug Seroquel was created to treat Schizophrenia; however, one of the side effects of this drug is drowsiness. It is currently being prescribed to treat insomnia, which is a side effect of stimulant ADHD drugs.

Several class action lawsuits have been filed because of the side effects of the continued use of these medications. There has already been a correlation discovered between the extended use of these stimulant drugs and the incidents of school violence that seem to be increasing each year.

In 1999, the Office of the Surgeon General conducted a survey entitled *Grading the Level of Evidence for Efficacy of Psychotropic Drugs in Children*. This survey addressed the short-term and long-term efficacy and safety of the most commonly prescribed drugs. The results of this survey revealed that only stimulants prescribed for ADHD, Selective Serotonin Reuptake Inhibitors (SSRI) prescribed for Obsessive-Compulsive Disorder (OCD), and Antipsychotics for Tourette's syndrome had two (2) or more randomized controlled trials (RCT's) for short-term efficacy. Also approved for short-term safety in two (2) or more RCT's were SSRI's for major depression, and Valproate and Carbamazepine for bi-polar and aggressive conduct disorders.

So how is "short term" defined? After checking the FDA webs site, Web MD, a medical dictionary, and several medical and naturopathic physicians, none were able to provide a definition for "short term" usage.

Some physicians believe the drugs should be taken every day, whether the child is in school or not. Other physicians will tell you to avoid giving the drugs to your child on weekends and over summer vacation. None of the psychologists that treated my son made any mention on whether he was to take the medication every day or only during the week when he was in school. I thought that since he was being given this prescription for inattention in school, that I should only give it to him on school days. It was through my own research that I discovered the damage it could do to brain function from the consistent high and crash the drug caused.

You, as the parent, will have to make the decision based on how your child reacts. Remember, these drugs are in the same category as cocaine. The drug takes effect, and the drug wears off – up and down. One minute your child is watching TV or doing homework, focused and absorbed in their task and all of the sudden, your child is bouncing off the walls, crying, frustrated because they can't get the right answer – and, if you are like most parents, you have no idea what happened because you weren't warned about what to expect when the drugs wear off. Is it safe for your child to be on this teeter-totter every day?

Of the listed categories of drugs - stimulants, SSRI's, Central Adrenergic Agonists, Valproate and Carbamazepine, Tricyclic Antidepressants, Benzodiazepines, Antipsychotics and Lithium - no long-term efficacy has been proven or even studied for that matter. Their efficacy is only assumed through clinical opinion, case reports, and uncontrolled trials. Within each of these categories of medications, along with the individual drugs prescribed within these categories, dangerous side effects have been reported.

The drug leaflets included with stimulant, SSRI, antidepressant, and other medications intended to affect the chemicals in the brain, list common side effects that may include:

☐ Insomnia

☐ Increased Blood Pressure

- ☐ Depression
- ☐ Anti-Social Behavior
- ☐ Thoughts of Suicide
- ☐ Thoughts of Hurting Yourself
- ☐ Mood Changes
- ☐ Skin Condition
- ☐ Allergic Reaction
- ☐ Fast, Pounding or Uneven Heartbeat
- ☐ Feeling Light-Headed or Fainting
- ☐ Headache
- ☐ Blurred Vision
- ☐ Joint Pain
- ☐ Jerky Muscles
- ☐ Diarrhea
- ☐ Vomiting
- ☐ Stomach Pain
- ☐ Menstrual Cramps
- ☐ Impotence
- ☐ Cough
- ☐ Dry Mouth
- ☐ Constipation
- ☐ Urinating Less or not at all
- ☐ Loss of Appetite
- ☐ Confusion
- ☐ Crying

- ☐ Irritable Temperament
- ☐ Aggression
- ☐ Restlessness
- ☐ Motor Tics or Twitches
- ☐ Hallucinations
- ☐ Weight Loss
- ☐ Weight Gain
- ☐ Trouble Concentrating
- ☐ Chest Pain
- ☐ Numbness and Seizure

Some stimulants have caused sudden death in children and adolescents with heart problems or congenital heart defects.

Warnings also advise: Avoid the use of stimulant medications if your child has used an MAO inhibitor, or if there is a history of glaucoma * tics or Tourette's syndrome * severe anxiety * overactive thyroid * liver disease * tension or agitation * high blood pressure * mental illness * psychotic disorder * bi-polar illness * depression or prior suicide attempt * epilepsy or seizure disorder * skin condition or history of alcohol or drug usage. Stimulant medications should be avoided if the individual is pregnant or nursing a baby. Long-term use has been shown to slow a child's growth. These drugs may impair vision or reactions.

**Be careful if you drive or do anything that requires you to be awake and alert. **

**Doesn't achieving success in school require a child to be awake and alert? **

A drug is approved by the FDA only for a defined population. Yet after its approval and market availability, physicians are at liberty to prescribe it for anyone, even though the drug company is only allowed to market the drug for the approved population (which typically is adults). Once drugs have reached the market for adults, pharmaceutical companies have fewer financial incentives to conduct expensive and demanding studies with children, to whom drugs may be given through off-label prescribing. The problem has been significant enough to press Congress into passing legislation.

The FDA Modernization Act of 1997 was created to provide financial incentives for drug sponsors to conduct research on previously approved and newly approved drugs that may provide a benefit to pediatric subjects.

Dr. Mark A. Riddle, director of Child and Adolescent Psychiatry at Johns Hopkins Hospital in Baltimore, MD, provided data at the 1999 annual meeting of the American Academy of Child and

Adolescent Psychiatry regarding *FDA Approved Pediatric Indications with Sufficient Data to Support Prescribing*. These medications were identified as:

- **Methylphenidate** (Ritalin),
- **Dextroamphetamine** (Dexedrine),
- **Pemoline** (Cylert) - all for children age 6 and over that have been diagnosed with ADHD.
- **Clomipramine** (Anafranil) - for children aged 10 and older that have been diagnosed with Obsessive-Compulsive Disorder.
- **Fluvoxamine** (Luvox) - for children aged 8 and over that have been diagnosed with Obsessive-Compulsive Disorder.
- **Sertralin**e (Zoloft) - for children aged 6 years and older that have been diagnosed with Obsessive-Compulsive Disorder; and,
- **Pimozid**e (Orap) - for children aged 12 and over for Tourette's syndrome.

Dr. Riddle also presented data regarding *FDA Approved Pediatric Indications without Sufficient Data to Support Prescribing*. The medications were identified as:

- **Amphetamine salts** (Adderall)
- **Dextroamphetamine** (Dexedrine) – for children aged 3 and over that have been diagnosed with ADHD
- **Chlorpromazine** (Thorazine) for bi-polar disorder, hyperactivity, or pervasive developmental disorder in children aged 6 months or older
- **Thioridazine** (Mellaril) and
- **Haloperidol** (Haldol) both for bi-polar disorder, hyperactivity, or pervasive developmental disorder for children 2 or 3 and over, respectively
- **Lithium carbonate** (Eskalith) for mania or **lithium carbonate** (Lithobid) for bi-polar disorder in children who are 12 and older
- **Diazepam** (Valium) for anxiety in children aged 6 months and over.

Finally, Dr. Riddle presented data regarding *Drugs with No FDA Approved Pediatric Indication but with Sufficient Data to Support Prescribing*. These drugs were identified as:

- **Bupropion** (Wellbutrin) and

- **Imipramine** (Tofranil) for ADHD in children aged 6 to 12 years
- **Desipramine** (Norpramin) for ADHD in children aged 7 to 13 years
- **Fluoxetine** (Prozac) for depression in children aged 8 to 17 years
- **Lithium** (Lithobid, Eskalith, Lithonate, Lithotabs) for aggression in hospitalized children aged 5 to 12 years
- **Haloperidol** (Haldol) for behavioral problems in children with Autism between the ages of 2 to 7 years
- **Naltrexone** (ReVia) for hyperactivity I in Autistic children aged 3 to 7 years old

The above information was presented in 1999. Since 1999, additional information regarding the safety of the above listed psychotropic medications along with newly approved medications prescribed to treat pediatric mental and behavioral disorders has been uncovered.

Between the years of 1990-2000 over 569 children were hospitalized, of those 380 were life threatening hospitalizations and 186 died. The 186 deaths were from the drug methylphenidate (Ritalin), as reported to the FDA Med Watch program, a voluntary reporting scheme, the numbers of which represent no more than 10% to 20% of the actual incidence.

In March of 2006, the FDA convened a Pediatric Advisory Committee to evaluate the cardiac adverse events and future cardiac risk of medications prescribed for ADD and ADHD. The committee found that there was significant risk and as a result, they went a step beyond their authority and recommended that all manufacturers of all medications used to treat these disorders includes an official "black box warning label" within the packaging to alert parents to this risk.

The FDA dismissed this panel without agreeing to follow their recommendations. One month later, the FDA convened a second Pediatric Advisory Committee with the same purpose. This second committee reached the same conclusions as the first committee.

Finally, in February of 2007, the FDA notified all manufacturers of these medications that they are now required to include a "black box warning label" in all packaging material. The FDA told manufacturers to revise the labels of the drugs to reflect concerns about the cardiovascular and psychiatric problems.

Draft versions of the guidelines were posted on the FDA web site and included discussion of reports of increased blood pressure and heart rate in ADHD patients, as well as cases of sudden death in some who have heart problems and heart defects. In adult patients, the reported problems also include stroke and heart attack.

The alerts also cover psychiatric problems, such as hearing voices, unfounded suspicions, and manic behavior, of which there is a slightly increased risk in patients who take the drugs. The guidelines also tell patients and their parents of precautions they can take to guard against the risks.

The FDA announced the order applies to the following 15 drugs:

- Adderall Tablets
- Adderall XR Extended-Release Capsules
- Concerta Extended-Release Tablets
- Daytrana Transdermal System
- Desoxyn Tablets
- Dexedrine Spansule Capsules and Tablets
- Focalin Tablets
- Focalin XR Extended-Release Capsules
- Metadate CD Extended-Release Capsules

- Methylin Oral Solution
- Methylin Chewable Tablets
- Ritalin Tablets
- Ritalin SR Sustained-Release Tablets
- Ritalin LA Extended-Release Capsules
- Strattera Capsule

Chapter 10

The Holistic Solution Begins with Nutrition

There are no established questionnaires or scales to diagnose any of these mental, emotional, or behavioral disorders on a holistic level. The diagnosis starts with identifying what, and how the specific behaviors are presenting in the young person's life. Followed by identifying when the problem started and what the normal response to the behavior has been, both at home and in the school environment?

Try to be less critical in this evaluation period. Avoid looking for problems when it may just be normal childhood behavior. It is often too easy to attach a label to a behavior instead of looking for an appropriate form of discipline or teaching your child how to take responsibility for their actions that may actually correct the problem. Sometimes just sitting down with your child and talking to them, without judgment, without anger, may provide the answers you are looking for.

One option is to begin your holistic approach by looking at the child's daily activities, including food intake and whether any behaviors manifest after eating certain types of foods. When the symptoms, behaviors, or actions you have observed are interfering in the daily life of your child it is time to involve the entire family in the finding the proper means to restore balance.

It is my belief that the majority of all physical imbalances are in some way tied to the food we eat. I wish I could say I had always thought that way. In fact, I can tell you that I was one of those people who believed that if it was for sale in the grocery store, it had to safe to eat. The idea that money could be a driving force behind the ingredients that are approved by the FDA never occurred to me. I ate and fed my family based on this clouded belief, until I started the nutrition class that was part of my Mind-Body Psychology program.

The instructor was actually finishing his last semester to be a naturopathic doctor, at the local naturopathic college. We began by learning about the difference between whole foods and processed foods, real nutrition vs chemically created vitamin and mineral supplements, and why artificial colors and flavors were added to foods. Did you know that "fresh" food in the grocery store has most likely already traveled for five or more days before it ever gets to the store? It is easy to get local, fresh food during the summer if there is a farmer's market in your neighborhood. But once the season is over, it is nearly impossible unless you live in California. At the time, I lived in Arizona and honestly, not much grows in the desert.

It was fall of 2004; Nick was off the drugs and because of that, he had just been transferred into the alternative school. I was trying to learn as much as I could about anything non-medical that would help him and in turn, help our family. With the knowledge on how the food industry works and the connection between the pharmaceutical industry and the food industry, I knew that I had to stop doing things the way I had been. Change is never easy though. At the time, I was just barely making ends meet even with the food stamp benefits I was getting. And I really had no idea how to change. I like cooking so the majority of our meals were eaten at home, but I cooked the way my mom had cooked. I made most of the same dishes mostly the same way she did. I had no idea there was another way. I wish the government division that sponsors the food stamp program would offer some type of shopping or cooking classes on how to choose and prepare healthy foods on a budget. I figured if Jamie Oliver could turn around an entire school district's food program without increasing their budget, someone would be able to do the same for moms like me. But there was nothing or no one back then. So, what I wanted to learn I had to research myself or ask some of my classmates. I have to tell you though, many of them were practicing a vegetarian lifestyle and my kids and I like meat. Yep, we are a family of carnivores or omnivores because I had no problem getting them to eat and like a lot of different vegetables, but meat still took center stage on the dinner plate.

I was raised with a set of taste buds aligned to the foods my mom fixed for us and my kids followed suit. But like I said, I had included a variety of fresh, raw, and cooked vegetables all along but packaged pasta and bottled or jar sauce, packaged helper meals, packaged side dishes, deli meats, chips, and soda made up the usual weekly menu. I honestly thought I was doing a decent job. I did eliminate some things, like processed cheese and most of the canned vegetables. I switched to fresh or frozen vegetables, except for the green beans. None of us really liked the taste of the frozen ones and fresh ones were out of my budget. As a little kid, I remember my dad having an awesome garden in our back yard every year. But he passed when I was 12 and I failed to pick up his garden magic – at least not in the containers that would fit on the patio or balcony of the apartment we lived in.

Between working full-time and going to school nights and weekends, I must admit I was into meals that were quick and easy to prepare. I felt rather good about getting rid of the canned goods, and Kool-Aid. The red dye #40 in the Kool-Aid really set my son off. I figured this out when I took a five day food diary home from school. At first I thought it was the sugar, but I had cut back to about half of what the packaged suggested. What I noticed was when I served the fruit punch flavor, within about 15-20 minutes he was either agitated or hyper. So, I got rid of the Kool-Aid and checked every label for Red dye 40.

I was reading every label on everything I bought, and I began to realize that there were artificial colors and flavors in about everything processed. I was slowing buying less and less processed foods, but there were still the cereals, helper meals, and other packaged goods. I was unable to go all organic at that time. So, I made the changes I could because my local grocery store offered a few organic brands priced equal to regular brand name products. I then turned my attention to what I was cooking and storing the food in.

Remember, that was more than 15 years ago and now most every grocery store has their own organic brand. In addition, Whole Foods has their "360" brand of reasonably priced organic food products.

I am not going to tell you or even suggest that you go into your kitchen and throw out all the processed foods and plastic ware. I did get rid of all the plastic food storage containers, once I found out that plastic was a hormone disrupter. I also switched from a microwave to a toaster oven. Now why would I get rid of the microwave you may be asking? I had read enough research on the radiation emitted, but more important to me was how it kills the nutrients in the food. I was just learning how nutrient deficient our food was to begin with because of the overplanting of commercial agricultural farms. I would like to see you do the same, but you need to do it your way. Let me explain a little more why I made that decision. I learned that when you put hot foods into plastic containers, some of that plastic leeches into the food. And, when you put plasticware in the microwave, you are actually cooking that plastic into whatever you are heating or cooking. Of course, I quickly learned that margarine was one molecule away from plastic. Country Crock was a staple at our table and in the food

I cooked. There are scientific studies that proved all of these statements to be true and I was convinced. Believe me I was reluctant to get rid of my plastic. I mean, I had three young kids that were kids you know? They rarely gave much thought to the things they handled. I was fairly sure there would be more than one occasion where I would be cleaning up broken glass. Nevertheless, I threw it all out. I know, you might be thinking I should have donated it to the Goodwill or the Salvation Army, right? It was a safety issue. If I eliminated it from my family's home, I had no intention of giving it to someone else. You know, do unto others and all that.

Cookware was another area that I had made changes in. Over the last couple of years, I had been shown reports that showed using cookware with a Teflon coating could lead to Alzheimer's. The reports explained that the coating was placed over an aluminum base and aluminum was proven to be a cause of disruptions in the neuro-pathways of the brain eventually leading to Alzheimer's disease. So, little by little, I had replaced all my cookware with stainless steel or cast iron.

Ok, so my cookware and storage dishes were good. Now it was time to tackle the food in the pantry. I can tell you, my two older kids totally believed I was playing favorites. Neither of them had ever presented any symptoms so they were unable to understand why I had to change things just for their brother. Have you ever tried to explain to teen and pre-teens that you are making changes for their own good? Yeah, well if you have you know that it is often in one ear and out the other. I decided to take things slow and that is what I would recommend to you too, especially if you have other kids.

Do you make out a menu for the meals you are going to prepare during the week? Yeah, me either. I found all kinds of reasons to avoid doing this. What I did discover is that it would have if I had given it a chance. Instead of shopping for the items I needed to prepare the meals on the menu, I went to the store and pretty much bought the same foods week after week and then tried to figure out what I could cook with what I had. I thought making out menus would take too much time, but when I look back now, I realize how much time and effort I actually wasted. I had more than enough resources to come up with meals, including a wide variety of cookbooks I could have used. I think it was simply another change and I was just unable to add one more at the time. Hopefully, you

have more "stick-to-itness" than I did. I know I could
have saved money and time if I had just invested the
effort in creating the menus before going to the store to
shop. Get the kids involved too. If they are old enough,
pick a night and let them cook. My boys have always
liked to cook, but my daughter never did. I found out
that they were more than willing to help with some
other chores if they got to cook too.

In the prior chapter, I shared the practice of using
kinesiology to check for food sensitivities. It is
possible that your child may have some type of
delayed food allergy which makes certain foods
unhealthy for them. The practice I described, where the
body leans forward or backward, you can easily teach
your children to do that. My kids loved to do it – and –
it took the "mean ole mommy" off my shoulders when
we were at the store. When my kids begged for
"goodies," I would have them hold the product in their
hands and ask their body if it was something that
would provide their bodies with the nutrients it needs
to keep working. They would simply say, "Is this good
for me?" and wait to see which way their body leaned
to know whether they could put it in the shopping cart
or whether it had to go back on the shelf. That means
mom is not the bad guy anymore.

Let the kids help when it comes to making out the grocery list. Besides, that is good training for when they are grown and need to shop on their own. Ask them what they would like to eat over the coming week and talk about why it might or might not be a good choice and if it is a good choice, what ingredients it takes to make it. Education is the best weapon for change. Kids absorb everything they see, hear, and feel for the first five or six years of their life – both good and bad. There are lots of good "food" movies out there I would highly recommend you watch with your kids. Movies like Food Matters; Super Size Me; Food, Inc.; and Thrive - not as foodie as the others but still a great movie.

Here is something you may be unaware of. School districts prepare the meals based on caloric intake instead of nutrition. The new push for healthier eating in schools has been transformed into higher carb and lower protein intake. The new program, "Healthy, Hunger-Free Kids Act," http://www.fns.usda.gov/school-meals/healthy-hunger-free-kids-act, focuses on fruits, vegetables, and whole grains. Sounds good right? Well not really. Take a look at the menu posted on your local school district's website. Breakfast for many of the elementary schools includes cold cereal, because the label says, "whole grain." I actually interviewed the person in charge of creating the menus for my local school district and was shocked at some of the answers I got. I asked about the cereal and was told it was "low-sugar" and whole grain. When I mentioned that the corn the cereal is made out of is more than likely genetically modified (GMO) and the whole grain is only whole before it is processed. She responded by saying, "Yes it is, it says so on the label." I just had to pause at that point. That response led me to ask whether anyone in the school lunch program was a certified nutritionist or had any training in that field. Her response, "No" really was no surprise unfortunately. She stated, "In my local school district, the employees in the school lunch program are contracted workers. They are union employees that work for a much larger corporation and have no real education in nutrition." I asked if there was an option for protein to be a bigger part of the menu because protein provides an extended period of attention and alertness; she said that protein holds a much smaller level of importance in the new food pyramid. I then asked whether any fresh, local foods were being purchased by the school district. She said that all of the elementary schools had heat and serve kitchens and most of the employees were moms that just needed or wanted a part time job and "did not have the skill level to work in a full kitchen." I found that curious, wondering if she understood that most of these moms were actually cooking meals for their families at home. She very proudly announced that every high school in the district is a Subway franchise. Yep, it seems school lunches are about the profit instead of the students. It is a business. The ala carte menu or ala carte bar is separate from the school lunch, and the Federal Government only reimburses for the main lunch. I was unable to find out how much the local schools are being reimbursed per meal, but she did say they were getting a $0.06 raise effect July 1, 2014. And she was really pleased with that. I am having trouble wrapping my head around how $0.06 could make that much of a difference.

The last thing I want is to overwhelm you with all this information, but I really do want to fire you up to take notice of what your children are eating and how it is affecting their ability to learn and just get through each day. Check out the Chef Ann Foundation. This group is making great strides in improving the quality of school lunches.

I am going to give you a few changes that you can make right away, beginning with the list of the Dirty Dozen fruits and vegetables – along with the Clean 15, which is updated annually. If you are unfamiliar with these lists, they rank conventionally grown fruits and vegetables that have the most (Dirty Dozen) and least (Clean 15) amount of pesticide residue on them when you buy them in the store. I used to think that I never had to worry about pesticides used in the growing process because I washed the fruits and vegetables I brought home. Unfortunately, I found out that when pesticides and herbicides are sprayed on a field it drips off the plants and soaks into the ground. Once in the soil, it is then absorbed inside of the plant through the root system. So even if you wash the outside, it is impossible to wash the inside of the fruit or vegetable. I would suggest that if you and your family likes what is on the Dirty Dozen list, either buy it organic. A simple fruit and vegetable cleaner is 1 part white vinegar to 2 parts clear water. Let them soak for 10-15 minutes and rinse them really good with clear water. Consider putting a filter system on your kitchen faucet. I have used the Pur Faucet Filter on my kitchen faucet for years and I have always been pleased with the results.

Now for the "Elephant in the Room" – and you knew I was going to go there – sugar. Despite what the commercials tell you, sugar is not sugar. Sugars are processed differently in the body. There are quite a few chemicals used in the process of turning sugar cane into white table sugar, including a bleaching process to make sure it is all pretty and white. The corn in high fructose corn syrup (HFCS) is made with GMO corn as is the corn syrup, corn starch, and corn flour.

In my kitchen, you will find organic raw cane sugar, raw honey, or 100% pure, organic maple syrup. I know agave syrup is used by many, but it is just not my preference. Beet sugar is a popular additive to many processed foods. Just know that around 85% of beet sugar made in the United States comes from GMO plants. If you are not baking, you can use Stevia leaf. Stevia can be grown in your garden and then dried for use at the table. The catch is that it is 300 times sweeter than sugar and some people say it leaves a bitter after-taste in their mouths. If you choose Stevia, make sure you buy it from an organic source and check for any added ingredients. Like most plants, Stevia is green so when you see a white powder, labeled Stevia, know that the leaves have been bleached to obtain the white color.

You may be thinking, "If I can't use regular sugar, I'll just go sugar-free." Please don't. The artificial sweeteners on the market are dangerous – plain and simple. Aspertame, the most common artificial sweetener used in food processing, is just one of many sweetening ingredients you might find on the labels you are now reading. Other names include Acesulfame K, Tagatose, Hydrogenated Starch Hydrolysates, Mannitol, Neotame, Polydextrose, Saccharin (made from petroleum), Sorbitol, and Sucralose (Splenda). Anything with "ose" or "tol" at the end is an artificial sweetener, including xylitol, which is actually a sugar alcohol (Dr. Oz Show, 2014). According to Dr. Boham, the use of artificial sweeteners actually shorts out the part of the brain that tells the body when it is satisfied. In return, the body tells the brain it needs to eat more and more in an attempt to reach that satisfaction point. That means more and more calories, more and more sugars in the blood and a greater risk of both obesity and diabetes down the road.

On his website, Dr. Mark Hyman (2014) really goes into the real causes of obesity and the evidence he uncovered that proves each statement to be true. I have picked out the more stand-out facts and listed them as follows:

1. The stuff America calls food is actually **biologically addictive**. No matter how much "willpower" you think you have, it is just a farce. Eating less and exercising more will lead to failure too because the body is programmed to actually shut-down when it gets less calories. His research revealed that in animal studies, rats work eight times harder to get sugar than they work to get cocaine. All calories are not the same, despite the Federal Governments protests that it is all about moderation. Scientific studies have proved that last statement false. Many of which are linked on Dr. Hyman's website.

2. There are a multitude of **addictive products** (nearly 600,000) within the food industry. More than that, they lie about the science behind it. Apparently sugar lights up the addiction center in the brain and that actually increases your cravings and hunger. Sugar calories are bad calories – really – because they put hunger in overdrive causing you to overeat and slow down your metabolism. Personal responsibility is important, but honestly, if you are truly addicted to the products the food

industry creates – what chance do you really have to succeed? Some food companies actually pay scientists, like David Allison (who received $2.5 million from Coke and Pepsi), to "debunk" the dangers of soda and junk food. Can we really expect someone being paid that kind of money to go against the company filling their pockets?

3. Have you ever heard the statement, "He's riding the fence"? It means someone is working both sides of a situation and refusing to commit to any one point of view. The **food environment is toxic**, and many 'medical experts' are doing exactly that. They pretend to be part of the solution while actually making us, the general public, sicker and fatter. From 2006 to 2011, the big companies that sell one quarter of the junk in America increased their sales from "healthier" products by $1.25 billion. While sales for higher sugar, higher calorie products also increased by $278 million in the same period.

4. The corruption from food industry money goes deep within our Government and "independent" professional organizations like

the American Nutrition and Dietetic Association (AND). The food industry "partnered" with Michelle Obama for her *Let's Move!* campaign and agreed to take 1.5 trillion calories out of the food supply. That may sound like a lot, but it is actually only 14 calories a day or one bite out of a Pop Tart. In taking something out, you know it is going to be replaced with something else. In this case, they add more low-fat, no-fat, or sugar-free lower calorie products (which still cause obesity and diabetes) and make Oreos 90 calories instead of 100. There is no scientific evidence anywhere that says that every American needs to drink at least three glasses of milk a day to get the recommended daily allowance (RDA) of calcium. To be honest, the scientists on the committees that advise the government often work for the industry. Can you say bias?? An 80-page summary of the dangers of sugar was completely left out of the final scientific report to the USDA, which makes up the guidelines. The Institute of Medicine, an independent group of scientists that advise the government on health matters has found their reports totally ignored. Believe it or not, the American Heart Association (AHA) gets $300,000 per endorsement of food products. That is why you see the AHA seal of approval on processed oat cereals with six different kinds of sugar. And the American Academy of Family Practice receives funding from Coke!

5. Did you know that you are actually 57% more likely to be overweight if your friends are overweight than if your parents are overweight. So much for blaming genetics. **Obesity and chronic disease (diabetes, heart disease, cancer) are contagious,** and the public campaigns are tainted with industry money – so who do we believe? How do we change this environment? One idea Dr. Hyman mentioned was starting community-based organizations that can create solutions to cure them. Dr. Hyman believes it is time to stop blaming the fat person and look at the real science behind why we are a fat nation (and increasingly, a fat world). He says we need to hold the food industry accountable, hold the government accountable and have truly independent science.

Who is left out there to believe? Have you ever seen the Facebook post that lists the member of Congress and the House of Representatives that have had prior affiliations with Monsanto? For me, this is all very disappointing. How do I raise my children up to trust our country's leaders if I am unable to trust them to be honest regarding their affiliations?

Additional research from many sources has shown that no matter what the age, each child diagnosed with a mental, emotional, or behavioral disorder exhibits these four commonalities:

- An adrenal imbalance
- An almost uncontrollable desire for sugar or carbohydrates
- Signs and symptoms of rapidly fluctuating blood sugar
- Multiple food sensitivities

Dr Ben Feingold, a professor of Allergy at the Kaiser Medical Center in San Francisco in 1973, presented a paper on food additives and hyperactivity in children to the American Medical Association. Dr. Feingold reported that the food habits of most Americans had changed in such a way that most people had come to rely on foods containing artificial ingredients. He cited a US Department of Agriculture report that only 3.3% of foods were prepared by the consumer from basic ingredients. The rest came from convenience foods processed by the food industry. The sheer magnitude of over 2700 intentional food additives as well as the amount of chemicals consumed on a daily basis compared with the numbers of children who suffer from hyperactivity and learning disabilities. He recommended that parent's limit processed food in favor of the fresh and natural.

Since Dr. Feingold's original report, more than 30 years have passed and yet the debate continues on whether a family's lifestyle plays a role in shaping children's health. Industrial representatives work hard blurring the relationship between their products and poor health. Every manufactured chemical has an industry behind it and reducing additives entails monetary loss.

Children today are exposed to hazards unknown just 30 years ago. Medical research is producing mounting evidence that exposure to environmental and chemical toxins can cause damage to the delicate brain growth of an unborn child during pregnancy. This type of neurological damage has the potential to cause learning disabilities, hyperactivity, and other child behavior disorders.

Continued exposure to identified chemical sources continues to grow as children are subjected to hundreds of different chemicals and neurotoxins simultaneously. These include chemical flavors and preservatives in food, pesticides in fruits and vegetables, chemicals in cleaning compounds, fabric softeners, cosmetics, and plastic, as well as vapors in vehicle exhaust, carpeting, paints, and upholstery.

Earlier I told you about the aluminum in the cookware I got rid of. Well, did you know there is aluminum in just about every antiperspirant on the store shelves? It is not in most of the products labeled as deodorants, but it is the primary ingredient in the antiperspirants. Your skin is the largest organ in your body and anything you put on it is absorbed right into your blood stream, and that of your kids. Chlorine is another big pollutant. It is in the water that comes out of our faucets so please do not drink tap water. Make the $20-$25 investment in a water filter if bottled water is out of your budget. In addition, replace the shower head with a shower filter to remove the chlorine from the water you and your kids shower with. Read the labels on the soaps, shampoos, crème rinses, and other personal hygiene products you buy. Sodium laurel sulphate and formaldehyde (remember dissecting those frogs in high school) are two primary ingredients – neither of which are good for you nor your body. Finally, find out if the water in your community has added fluoride. If so, make sure your water filter removes it. If you are feeding your kids healthy foods, there is no need for fluoride in their toothpaste in order for them to have strong, healthy teeth and gums.

Chapter 11
Genetically Modified Ingredients

The debate has broadened to include Genetically Modified foods. Genetic Engineering (GE) or Genetic Modification (GM) is the laboratory process of artificially manipulating or inserting genes into the DNA of food crops or animals. The result is called a genetically modified organism or GMO. Genetic Modified Organisms can be created with genes from bacteria, viruses, insects, animals or even humans.

The majority of Americans surveyed state they would not eat GMOs if labeled, but unlike most other industrialized countries, labeling is optional in the United States and Canada.

Genetically modified foods are most commonly used to refer to crop plants created for human or animal consumption using the latest molecular biology techniques. These plants are modified in the laboratory to enhance desired traits such as increased resistance to herbicides or improved nutritional content.

The enhancement of desired traits was traditionally done through breeding; however, conventional plant breeding methods can be very time consuming and are often not very accurate. Genetic engineering can create plants with the exact desired trait very rapidly and with great accuracy. For example, plant geneticists can isolate a gene responsible for drought tolerance and insert that gene into a different plant. The new genetically modified plant will gain drought tolerance as well. Not only can genes be transferred from one plant to another, but genes from non-plant organisms also can be used.

The prevalence of genetically modified foods in U.S. grocery stores is more widespread than is commonly thought. While there are very few genetically-modified whole fruits and vegetables available on produce stands, highly processed foods, such as vegetable oils and breakfast cereals, most likely contain some percentage of genetically-modified ingredients because the raw ingredients have been pooled into one processing stream from many diverse sources. Also, the presence of soybean derivatives as food additives in the modern American diet virtually ensures that all U.S. consumers have been exposed to genetically modified food products.

Genetically modified plants currently available in the United States include:

1. Cotton – As of 2020, approximately 96% of cotton grown is genetically modified. Although it may be unclear as to why this plant is on this list, it is important to remember that cotton is used to create cottonseed oil, which is an ingredient in many processed foods, as well as for animal feed.

2. Papaya – Nearly all of the Hawaiian papaya seed has been genetically modified, since 1998, in an attempt to protect papaya plants from the ringspot virus.

3. Soy – Since 1996, GMO soy has been used as animal feed, food products, and food preservatives. As of 2020, nearly 94% of soy is genetically modified.

4. Sugar Beets – Nearly 99.9% of sugar beet products, as of 2020, are made with genetically modified seed.

5. Yellow Summer Squash and Zucchini – The first squash were genetically modified in 1995; however, it is believed that only about 10% of squash for sale has been genetically modified.

6. Corn – As of 2020, 92% of corn grown is genetically modified. GMO corn is grown in every state at any given time according to the

USDA. GMO corn is used in processed foods and drinks as well as in feed for CAFO cows and chickens.

7. Golden Rice – Modified to include Vitamin A to address blindness and potential death caused by Vitamin A deficiency.

8. Rapeseed – or Canola oil is used for cooking and as a food ingredient. Data from 2020 reports that 95% of rapeseed is grown from GMO seed.

9. Animal feed – A variety of GMO crops are used as 'vegetarian' feed for animals raised in Confined Animal Feed Operations (CAFO) who are then slaughtered and end up in the meat department of our grocery stores.

10. Patents have been filed for the creation of genetically modified Potatoes, Apples, Alfalfa, and Pink Pineapples. The actual percentage of these crops sold to the general public is unknown.

11. Salmon & Pigs – AquAdvantage Salmon and GalSafe Pigs are available to consumers, they have been approved for sale and human consumption. Farm raised salmon are fed

artificially colored feed and paint chips to
modify the 'flesh color' of the fish.

Most concerns about genetically modified foods
fall into three categories: environmental hazards,
human health risks, and economic concerns.

There are three categories of genetically modified
(GM) foods: crops, dairy products and meat, and
enzymes and additives created from genetically
modified bacteria and fungus. Not everyone who
conscientiously avoids genetically modified foods
chooses to be strict in all categories.

U.S. dairy products may contain milk from cows
injected with rbGH (recombinant bovine growth
hormone). And both meat and dairy products usually
come from animals that have eaten genetically
modified feed.

Genetically modified bacteria and fungi are used in
the production of enzymes, vitamins, food additives,
flavorings, and processing agents in thousands of foods
on the grocery shelves as well as health supplements.
Aspartame, the artificial sweetener, is a product of
genetic engineering.

Foods that may contain genetically modified soy or
corn derivatives or genetically modified vegetable oil
include: infant formula, salad dressing, bread, cereal,

hamburgers and hot dogs, margarine, mayonnaise, crackers, cookies, chocolate, candy, fried food, chips, veggie burgers, meat substitutes, ice cream, frozen yogurt, tofu, tamari, soy sauce, soy cheese, tomato sauce, protein powder, baking powder, alcohol, vanilla, powdered sugar, peanut butter, enriched flour and pasta. Non-food items include cosmetics, soaps, detergents, shampoo, and bubble bath.

Genetic engineering is used in the production of many food additives, flavorings, vitamins, and processing aids, such as enzymes. These ingredients said to improve the color, flavor, texture, and aroma of foods and to preserve, stabilize, and add nutrients to processed foods. Among vitamins, vitamin C (ascorbic acid) is often made from corn; vitamin E is usually made from soy. Vitamins A, B2, B6, and B12 may be genetically modified as well. Both Vitamin D and Vitamin K may have carrier ingredients derived from genetically modified corn sources, such as starch, glucose, and maltodextrin. In addition to finding these vitamins in supplements, they are sometimes used to fortify foods. Organic foods, even if fortified with vitamins, are not allowed to use ingredients derived from genetically modified substances. Flavorings can also come from corn or other genetically modified sources. For example, "hydrolyzed vegetable protein (HVP), a commonly used flavor enhancer derived from corn and soy as well as Vanillin could be genetically modified.

The correlation between proper nutrition and behavioral disorders has presented a challenge for scientific study. The biggest problem is that children rarely react to food additives, genetically modified ingredients, or chemical additives in the exact same way.

Everyday diet should be one of the first things that a practitioner looks at when trying to determine the cause of a child's mental, emotional or behavioral disorder. The following questions should be asked:

1. Is the child eating at regular intervals?
2. Is the child drinking enough fluids?
3. Is the child eating whole foods or convenience foods?

It is not necessary to clean out the pantry to affect a wholesome diet change. Simply make a list the next time you go to the store and buy non-GMO foods and organic vegetables. If cost is a factor, start by picking out a few of your favorite foods and look for brands that do not use GM ingredients. Little by little, your tastes and that of your family will adjust to the healthier foods and you will find that you no longer crave foods that your body knows is unable to provide the nutrition it needs.

You can avoid Genetically Modified foods by buying organic, looking for foods labeled non-GMO and staying away from foods that contain the top four GM ingredients – corn, soy, canola oil, and cottonseed oil.

Genetically modified livestock, fowl, and fish have not been approved for human consumption in the U.S. However, many are raised on GM feed and grains. While shopping, look for grass-fed / grass-finished or regeneratively raised meat and wild caught fish. The following companies produce non-GMO eggs:

Egg Innovations Organic
Eggland's Best Organic
Land O'Lakes Organic
Nest Fresh Organic
Organic Valley
Pete and Jerry's Organic Eggs
Wilcox Farms Organic

Genetically modified organisms have found their way into the following foods:

Alternative Meat Products

Dairy Products

Alternative Dairy Products

Baby Foods & Infant Formula (Beech-Nut has an organic line of baby food products is seeking verification for all of their products from the Non-GMO Project)

Grains, Beans & Pasta

Cereals & Breakfast Bars

Baked Goods

Frozen Foods

Soups, Sauces & Canned Foods

Condiments, Oils, Dressings & Spreads

Snack Foods

Candy, Chocolate Products & Sweeteners

Sodas, Juices & Other Beverages

Many processed foods contain ingredients that are derived from genetically modified organisms. Look for the following ingredients on the package before you buy it.

Aspartame

baking powder

caramel color

cellulose

citric acid

cobalamin

corn gluten

corn masa

corn oil

corn syrup

cornmeal

cornstarch

cyclodextrin

cystein

dextrin

dextrose

diacetyl

diglyceride

fructose

glucose

glutamate

glutamic acid

gluten

glycerides

glycerin

glycerol

glycine

hemicelluloses

high fructose corn syrup (HFCS)

hydrogenated starch

hydrolyzed vegetable protein

inositol

invert sugar

isoflavones

lactic acid

lecithin

leucine

lysine

malitol

maltodextrin

maltose

mannitol

methylcellulose

milo starch

modified starch

monosodium glutamate (MSG)

oleic acid	phenylalanine
phytic acid	sorbitol
soy flour	soy isolates
soy lecithin	soy protein starch
stearic acid inverse syrup	tempeh
threonine	tocopherols (Vitamin E)
tofu	trehalose
triglyceride	vegetable fat
vegetable oil	Vitamin B12
Vitamin E	xanthan gum

Many brands have proudly posted their intent to go GMO-free, or they have always been GMO-free. Some brands you may or may not be aware of include:

1. Whole Foods – 365 Everyday Value brand
2. Amy's Kitchen – all-natural soups and chili's
3. Annie's Organic Homegrown Foods – 50+ varieties
4. Ciao Bella Gelato – 20 varieties of sorbet
5. Finn Crisp – 6 varieties of rye crispbread
6. Glee Gum – Chewing gum
7. Post Cereal – Grape Nuts
8. Hodgson Mill – 80+ products
9. Jolly Time – 7 varieties of popcorn

10. Kashi – 21 varieties of cereal

11. Kettle – All flavors of potato chip

12. Kind – Healthy grain bars – 9 varieties currently certified GMO-free with 19 others in the process

13. Murray's Chicken – naturally raised, antibiotic free, certified humane and GMO-free

14. Organic Valley – All of their dairy products

15. Weetabix – British breakfast biscuits

Dr. Abram Hoffer pioneered megavitamin research and treatment back in the early 1950's, and more than half a century later, the medical profession still largely ignores the results of his study. Hoffer and his colleagues conducted the first double-blind controlled vitamin trials in psychiatric history in 1952. He was among the first to employ vitamin C as an antioxidant, use the B-vitamins against heart disease, and, with Dr. Humphrey Osmond, was the first to employ niacin to treat behavioral disorders.

Finding vitamins that can be readily absorbed by the body is important. Formulas that are in liquid form are taken sublingually, as well as natural juices or teas that are made with natural ingredients (like wheat grass and herbal teas) are more nutritionally available than commercial vitamins produced by pharmaceutical companies. If you choose to use a commercial multivitamin/mineral formula, take one of the tablets or capsules and place it in about one cup of room temperature water. Wait approximately 20 minutes and then make note of how much of the pill or capsule has dissolved. The amount dissolved is fairly equivalent to the amount being absorbed by the body. The remainder of the pill or capsule will usually pass through the digestive system and be eliminated.

Have each member of the entire family complete a 5-day food diary, you will get a great overall view of how healthy your family really is eating, and you may just pick up on some food sensitivities. The food diary asks the person to note how they felt within a two hour window of eating. Sit down together and talk about what the food diary is saying about each person. Schedule regular mealtimes for the entire family and involve the whole family in shopping for and preparing meals as often as you can.

Chapter 12

Natural Therapy Alternatives

History has proven the effective use of plant medicines. In Traditional Chinese Medicine (TCM), Ayurvedic Medicine and Native American Medicine plants have been used for over 5,000 years to restore and maintain balance in the body. Science is just beginning to understand what herbalists, village medicine men/women and healers have known for eons, that plants provide natural options that rarely include side effects for the treatment of disease.

The debate is in the use of whole plant or through a "standardized" formula that can be patented and made into a pharmaceutical product. Herbs carry a wide variety of healing constituents in their leaves, stems, flowers, and roots. Knowing which part of the plant to use as well as the dosage and length of treatment is particularly important. To ensure you are safely using herbal remedies, either consult someone trained in the practice of herbalism or, if you prefer to self-treat, make sure you have used a variety of sources to get your information. There are thousands of herb books on the market, however, there are much less that have actually been written by individuals who are trained or have worked with these plants for many, many years. Companies like Rodale put out a variety of books on natural therapies, but no information is available on whether the individual(s) writing those books has the educational background to be making those recommendations or is doing anything more than just rewriting information from another source. I recommend the following herbalist resources for herbal medicine books, include Matthew Wood, Rosemary Gladstar, David Hoffman, Leslie Tierra, and Susan Weed, to name a few. All of these sources are highly qualified in the practice of herbalism. Another thing to keep in mind, each herbalist has their personal preferences regarding the herbs and blends they use for specific treatments. This is why I suggest you read at least three books by three different authors. You may find that you resonate with the information presented by one author more than the others, and that is ok. There are also a variety of herbal programs available, should you want your education to go deeper into the study than you can glean from personal reading. As I mentioned earlier, I attended the Southwest Institute of Healing Arts in Tempe, AZ to get my associate's in Western Herbalism and at this writing, A few years later, I attended the American College of Healthcare

Sciences, graduating from their master's program in Complementary and Alternative Medicine. Most recently, I graduated from the Energetic Health Institute with a certificate in holistic nutrition. Several of the herbalists mentioned above have their own training programs. If you choose to go that route, check into several programs and go with the one that truly resonates within.

When plants are used for medicinal purposes, either as a whole plant or the essential oils produced, the practice is called Phytotherapy (Penoel, 1999). The use of essential oils (plant volatile oils) goes back over 4000 years to the Egyptian civilization. These oils were used most commonly as part of the burial tradition for royal families. Greek physicians traveling through Egypt brought the use of these oils back to Greece with them. Records dating back to the time of Hippocrates document the medicinal use of these oils.

As a recognized medical therapy, general practitioners or medical specialists in Europe must either complete a basic training program or the full three year education program. In France, they practice the use of essential oils as phytotherapists. As these oils are up to 300 times more potent than a cup of herbal tea, it is important that the person recommending or using these oils has been educated on the correct way to use them. The Institute of Aromatic Medicine states: "Persons using aromatology (the practice of using essential oils for medical purposes) must be one of the following:

8.5.1 An accountable member, i.e., a health care professional who is a member of an aromatology association, or

8.5.2 A health care assistant, i.e., a health care professional who has attended an introductory program on aromatherapy of at least two days if external to the hospital plus extra tuition by the accountable member, or a health care professional who has attended an introductory program on aromatherapy of at least two days run by an accountable member.

There are specific contraindications or times the use of essential oils should be avoided. Make sure you have consulted a practitioner who has education and experience using these oils or do your own research. If you choose to do your own research, find several sources that have been written by registered aromatherapists, medical practitioners, or science based resources. Do not take the word of the manufacturer of the oils you are buying. They may or may not be accurate in their recommendations, but you can rest assure they will tell you what you want to hear in order to sell their oils. Remember, even the American Heart Association can be bought. They lend their name to otherwise unhealthy products for a fee. So, if there is monetary consideration that goes to the author, seek other sources.

Compared to the use of herbs and essential oils, flower essence therapy is the baby considering it has only been around since the early 20th century. Dr. Edward Bach, from the United Kingdom, believed that most illness had a deeper, emotional connection to both the creation and the healing of the disease. His research turned to the "essence" or living spirit of the plants and flowers. To capture that essence, Dr. Bach placed the flowers or plants in glass bowls of clear spring water, in the sunlight, allowing the energy from the sun to permeate through the flower or plant into the water in the bowl. I have used flower essences myself, during extremely stressful times in my life. I created a specific blend to help my son when he was so emotionally distraught over his lack of success in the public school environment. And I have witnessed how these essences literally brought a friend of mine back from the brink of suicide following the death of her son. I honestly believe in the use of these essences especially for young people who are under emotional stress or demonstrate anxiety or phobias. There have been no contraindications noted for the use of flower essences. It should be noted, however, that the essences may contain an alcohol base (often brandy) as a preservative. The amount is minimal, but it is important that you are aware of this.

Just like in allopathic medicine, no one treatment is right for every person, so I am offering you the information I have gleaned from years of study, personal use, and use with my son and clients on three of the most commonly used natural therapies. You may end up choosing to go with a single type of therapy or you may choose to combine two or all three with the allopathic medicine you are currently using. If you choose to replace the pharmaceuticals you or your child is taking, talk to a doctor and do it safely. Remember, these are highly addictive drugs and if your child has been taking them regularly for a number of years, they need to be weaned out of the body. Whatever your choice, do it safely. Seek help from someone you trust.

All of the following natural therapies address the body's need to return to homeostasis or balance. The information is divided up by the disorders commonly diagnosed in childhood.

The following herbal remedies are known to address **Stress and Anxiety Disorders** and can be taken alone or in combination with other herbs.

Amalaki- Emblica officinalis: In Ayurvedic Medicine, Amalaki is said to restore balance to the three constitutional elements, or doshas, that control life, as well as provide an abundance of antioxidant benefits. Amalaki is believed to contain adaptogenic properties. Adaptogens are nontoxic in normal doses, produce a nonspecific defensive response to stress, and have a normalizing influence on the body. They normalize the hypothalamic-pituitary-adrenal axis and form a new class of natural metabolic regulators that affect muscle and fat mass, glucose sensitivity and cardiac function. Adaptogens have a normalizing effect on the body and are capable of either toning down the activity of hyperfunctioning systems or strengthening the activity of hypofunctioning systems.

Bacopa- Bacopa monnieri: In Ayurvedic medicine, Bacopa is considered a main rejuvenating herb for nerve and brain health. Bacopa contains both saponins and flavonoids. Saponins are glycosides of steroids, steroid alkaloids (steroids with a nitrogen function) or triterpenes found in plants. Bacosapins provide antidepressant and antioxidant protection, which in turn fight free radicals produced during times of stress. Flavonoids are known for their antioxidant activity, which also fight free radicals.

California Poppy- Eschscholzia californica: California Poppy contains alkaloids that provide sedative properties that alleviate anxiety, restlessness, and insomnia. Alkaloids are a naturally occurring amine produced by a plant and are usually derivatives of amino acids.

Eleuthero- Eleutherococcus senticosus: The saponins in Eleuthero support the adrenal medulla by balancing the secretion of epinephrine/norepinephrine to facilitate blood flow to the brain. Eleuthero is an adaptogen, which increases the body's resistance to stresses such as trauma, anxiety, and bodily fatigue.

Licorice – Glycyrrhiza glabra: The saponins in Licorice support the adrenal cortex in response to adrenocartiocotropic hormone (ACTH) which influences the body's reaction to stress and emotions. Licorice is an adaptogen.

Linden – Tilia spp: The flowers of the Linden tree contain a high concentration of active compounds. These compounds create a nervine response in the Central Nervous System which acts as a mild sedative that eases nervous tension, restlessness, and hysteria.

Oats - Avena sativa: Oat seed has been prescribed as a restorative nerve tonic for a wide range of nervous conditions, including nervous anxiety, worry, depression and insomnia. Oats are thought to gently raise energy levels and support an over stressed nervous system.

Periwinkle - Vinca minor: Periwinkle's indole alkaloids improve cerebral arterial activity and oxygen consumption, which enhances blood circulation and metabolism in the brain.

Rhodiola- Rhodiola rosea: Rhodiola has been proven to be very effective for improving mood and alleviating depression. Russian research shows that it improves both physical and mental performance and reduces fatigue. As an adaptogen, Rhodiola's effects are attributed to its ability to optimize serotonin and dopamine levels in the brain.

Skullcap – Scutellaria laterifolia: Skullcap's nutritive qualities ease nervous exhaustion, depression, agitation, and anxiety. Skullcap has been used traditionally as a mild sedative in the form of herbal teas, tablets, and capsules. The aqueous (water) extract of the flowering parts have been traditionally used by Native Americans as a nerve tonic and for its sedative and diuretic properties. The anxiolytic properties of skullcap have also been shown to be as useful in the treatment of anxiety disorders as antidepressants such as the class of selective serotonin reuptake inhibitors (SSRI's).

When the body is under stress, the adrenal glands that sit on top of each kidney release a series of stress hormones. Each adrenal gland has two parts, the adrenal medulla, and the adrenal cortex. The adrenal medulla releases the hormones epinephrine and norepinephrine – the "speed" hormones. They increase the heartbeat and respiration, enhance blood sugar levels by converting glycogen to glucose in the liver, and can raise blood pressure. The adrenal cortex is responsible for certain behavioral actions, regulates metabolism, the immune system, and several other body functions through the release of cortisol and hydrocortisone. The cortex also releases a hormone that balances the amount of sodium and potassium the kidneys secrete. The other hormones secreted from the adrenal cortex are actually synthesized from cholesterol. They enhance the breakdown of proteins especially those responsible for creating inflammation in the body and even influence the emotional response to the stressor.

Young people are often thought to be stress-free when in fact they are often exposed to stressors equal to or greater than the adults in their life. Excess stress causes adrenal depletion and the release of an overload of the stress hormones which can lead to inflammation, early onset diabetes, obesity, and otherwise unexplainable behavioral changes.

Herbs for **Nutrition, Cleansing and Eating Disorders** can be taken alone or in combination with other natural therapies:

Alfalfa - Medicago sativa: Alfalfa has been used for digestive system issues for over 400 years. As a nourishing tonic, alfalfa contains eight essential amino acids, natural Vitamin K, beta-carotene, and fluoride. It clears toxins, promotes appetite and weight gain. It neutralizes acids and poisons and has a natural ability to stimulate the pituitary gland, hardens bones naturally and can absorb and carry intestinal waste from the body.

Amalaki- Emblica officinale: Amalaki fruit contains the highest natural source of Vitamin C. It is rich in bioflavonoids and flavones, which provide the pigment in fruits and vegetables and polyphenols, which provide antioxidant benefits. In Ayurvedic Medicine, Amalaki is said to revitalize the organs of the body and balance blood glucose levels.

Burdock – Arctium lappa: Burdock is an alterative that promotes blood and lymph cleansing and is a reliable source of nutrients. It promotes the elimination of metabolic waste, promotes kidney function, aids in the metabolism of carbohydrates and supports the function of the pituitary gland by maintaining hormonal balance. Alteratives have blood-purifying qualities that enhance glandular, liver, kidney, spleen and bowel function by speeding tissue restoration. These herbs promote the flow of bile aiding digestion and fights against constipation, and they contain nutrients necessary to achieving and maintaining good health.

Cleavers – Galium aparine: Cleavers is an alterative that facilitates the removal of catabolic wastes in the lymphatic and glandular body systems. Cleavers are known as the best overall tonic for nutrient support.

Chlorella – Chlorella contains all the vitamins including B, C, E, Zinc, Calcium, Copper, Magnesium, Iron, Germanium, Protein (60%). Chlorella is a single-celled, fresh water green algae and is reported to help with stress, healthy gums, bad breath, digestion, and elimination. It is an excellent detoxifier of heavy metals including cadmium, lead, mercury, and copper. Chlorella increases sustained energy and immune system health.

Essential Fatty Acids - EFA's are fatty acids that cannot be constructed within an organism from other components by any known chemical pathways; and therefore, must be obtained from the diet. Unfortunately, the Standard American Diet (SAD) is considerably higher in Omega 6 EFAs, called arachidonic acid and linoleic acid, than it is in the Omega 3 EFA, or the alpha-linolenic acid (ALA). ALA is readily found in green leafy vegetables, fish, phytoplankton, and algae. EFA's are responsible for carrying the fat soluble A, D, E and K vitamins.

Gymnema - Gymnema sylvestris: In Ayurvedic Medicine, gymnema was reportedly successful in controlling the blood sugar level without reducing it to below the normal range. It blocks the taste of sugar and the passages that sugar is normally absorbed through. Gymnema will not affect the flavor of food, but it will reduce those sugar cravings.

Hops – Humulus lupulus: Dried female buds of the hops plant have a high methylbutenol content, which has a mild sedative effect on the central nervous system. Hops have bitter attributes improving appetite and digestion. It is an excellent source of niacin and tones the stomach muscles, cleans the liver, and increases bile flow.

Lecithin - The soy phosphotides in Lecithin are reported to aid in the lowering of both cholesterol and triglyceride levels in the blood. Lecithin is an integral part of cell membranes, and can be totally metabolized, so it is virtually non-toxic to humans. When adding lecithin to the supplements you are taking, make sure you are buying an organic form as lecithin is most commonly a soy derivative and most soy comes from genetically modified sources. I typically buy organic sunflower lecithin.

Oats - Avena sativa: Oat seed acts as a restorative nerve tonic and eases nervous anxiety, worry, depression and insomnia. It improves appetite along with thyroid and estrogen deficiencies.

Rosehips - Rosa canina: Rose hips are used in teas, tonics, and jams. They are high in Vitamins A, C (more than sixty times that of citrus juice) and E, bio-flavonoids, and other bioactive compounds. It is also a fairly good source of essential fatty acids.

Spirulina- Spirulina plantensis: This one-celled plankton contains beta carotene, A, B2, B6, D, E, K, potassium, calcium, zinc, magnesium, selenium, iron, folic acid, all nine amino acids, and has twenty-six times the calcium of milk. Spirulina energizes the brain, helps satisfy hunger naturally and balances blood sugar levels.

These natural remedies are known to address **Memory, Learning, Concentration and Attention Disorders** and can be taken alone or in combination with other herbs:

Bacopa- Bacopa monnieri: In Ayurvedic medicine, Bacopa is considered a main rejuvenating herb for nerve and brain health. Bacopa contains both flavonoids and saponins. The Bacosides play a protective role in the synaptic functions of the nerves in the brain. Bacopa also improves protein synthesis and the oxidation of fats in the blood, especially in brain cells, which is said to contribute to increased intelligence and memory.

Eleuthero- Eleutherococcus senticosus: The saponins in Eleuthero support the adrenal medulla by supporting the secretion of adrenalin/noradrenalin to facilitate blood flow to the brain.

Foti- Polygonum multiflorum: In Traditional Chinese Medicine, Foti is thought to enhance learning and memory and prevent the degeneration of nigrostriatal dopaminergic neurons (source of dopamine) in the brain. Foti roots contain considerable amounts of lecithin and stilbene glycosides with superior antioxidant activity.

Ginkgo – Ginkgo biloba: Ginkgo contains flavone glycosides, which enhance the uptake of oxygen and glucose to the brain and prevent free radical damage to the cells. The use of ginkgo biloba for memory enhancement, increased attention span and to alleviate feelings of depression has been used for centuries in Traditional Chinese Medicine. Ginkgo, also called Maidenhair Tree, is the oldest species of tree on the Earth. It is the only tree that survived the Hiroshima atomic blast and is still alive today.

Gotu kola – Centella asiatica: In Ayurvedic Medicine, Gotu kola is considered a rejuvenator herb and has been used for centuries to enhance learning and memory. Two main active constituents in Gotu kola are Bacoside A and B. Bacoside A assists in release of nitric oxide that allows the relaxation of the aorta and veins, to allow the blood to flow more freely through the body. Bacoside B is a protein attributed to nourishing the brain cells. Gotu kola is used to revitalize the brain and nervous system, increase attention span and concentration, and combat aging. Gotu kola has antioxidant properties.

Hawthorn – Crataegus laevigata: Hawthorn is a nutritive herb that has restorative properties for blood vessels and improves blood flow to the brain.

Hyssop – Hyssopus officinalis: The active constituents in Hyssop's volatile oil relax peripheral blood vessels helping to increase alertness.

Licorice – Glycyrrhiza glabra: The saponins in Licorice support the adrenal cortex in response to adrenocartiocotropic hormone (ACTH) which influences the body's reaction to stress and emotions.

Rhodiola- Rhodiola rosea: As an adaptogen, Rhodiola's effects are attributed to its ability to optimize serotonin and dopamine levels in the brain subsequently improving work performance, mood, mental clarity, memory, and attention span. In one study, the Rhodiola rosea group decreased proofreading errors by 88% while the control group increased proofreading errors by 84%.

Rosemary – Rosmarinus officinalis: Rosemary is historically known as the "herb of remembrance." The active terpene alcohols and the compound cineole in Rosemary make this herb a valuable addition to any formula to relieve brain fog, memory problems, and depression.

The following natural remedies are known to

address **Nervousness, Hyperactivity, Insomnia and Specific Psychological Disorders** and can be taken alone or in combination with other herbs:

Catnip – Nepeta cataria: Catnip contains volatile oils, sterols, acids, and tannins. The primary terpene, nepetalactone, provides a mild sedative action that relieves nervous agitation and hyperactivity.

Chamomile – Matricaria recutita: Chamomile's volatile oils serve as a calming sedative/relaxant and relieve restlessness, irritability, moodiness, and nervous stomach.

Hyssop – Hyssopus officinalis: Hyssop is a gently relaxing nerve tonic suitable for treating nervous exhaustion, overwork, anxiety, and depression.

Lavender – Lavendula officinalis: Lavender contains the terpene alcohol, linalol, a type of aromatic or volatile oil. Lavender eases nervous irritability and promotes relaxation.

Lemon Balm – Melissa officinalis: The volatile oils in Lemon Balm emit a pleasant aroma and flavor. This herb acts as a mild relaxant easing nervousness.

Linden – Tilia spp: The flowers of the Linden tree contain a high concentration of active compounds. These compounds create a nervine response in the Central Nervous System which acts as a mild sedative that eases nervous tension, restlessness, and hysteria.

Oats - Avena sativa: Oat seed has been used as a restorative nerve tonic for a wide range of nervous conditions, including nervous anxiety, worry, depression and insomnia.

Passionflower – Passiflora incarnate: Passionflower leaves and roots have a long history of use among Native Americans in North America. Passionflower has been found to contain beta-carboline harmala alkaloids which are MAOIs with anti-depressant properties. These alkaloids have calmative and sedative properties which allay nervousness and promote rest, natural sleep and help alleviate insomnia and nightmares.

Peppermint – Mentha piperita: The volatile oils in peppermint provide a gentle pick me up, enhances circulation and secretions in the stomach which relieves nausea caused by a nervous stomach.

Skullcap – Scutellaria laterifolia: Skullcap has been used traditionally as a mild sedative in the form of herbal teas, tablets, and capsules. The aqueous (water) extract of the flowering parts have been traditionally used by Native Americans as a nerve tonic and for its sedative and diuretic properties.

St. John's Wort- Hypericum perforatum: St. John's Wort is commonly known for its ability to alleviate mild depression due to the primary constituent hypericin, which is a glycoside. St. John's Wort also has properties that make it safe as a sedative nervine.

HERBAL ACTIONS

If you are just learning about herbs you might be confused by some of the terms used within the herb section you just read. Hopefully, this next section will clarify any questions you might have. The terms are simply listed alphabetically for ease of use.

Adaptogen herbs are considered intelligent herbs. These building herbs strengthen the hypothalamus-pituitary-ovarian (HPO) axis and just seem to 'know' which part of the body needs the most help. Taken over time they build up your overall health and wellness and help you have more of a resiliency to the negative effects of stress.

Not all adaptogens are created equal. Each herb has its own specific indications and herbal energetics that are better suited for one person or another. Especially when these herbs are matched to you from an energetic perspective these are safe plants that can be taken in larger quantities for an extended period of time.

Alterative herbs support specific elimination pathways of the body. Depending on their specific action they may clear a congested liver, encourage urination, support the lungs for increased breath (and release of CO_2), open the pores in the skin, move the lymph, and move the bowels. Alterative herbs are often used for problems such as constipation, eczema, acne, boils, etc.

Herbs in this category are generally safe but if used too aggressively or for a prolonged period of time they can create an imbalance and potentially create a dependence like you might find with a pharmaceutical.

Anodyne herbs ease the sense of pain. Anodyne herbs can be completely safe, or they can be low-dose botanicals that should never be used beyond one or two drops. Herbs may also have a special affinity for diverse types of pain as some herbs are better suited to nervous system pain while others have an affinity for muscle pain.

Anti-inflammatory herbs work in a variety of ways to lessen the inflammatory response in the body. When a glossary term contains the word "anti" it lets us know WHAT it does but rarely does this classification break herbs down into HOW it actually works.

Antimicrobial herbs can be useful against viral infections, bacterial and fungal infections.

Antispasmodic herbs affect the nervous system to relieve muscle tension and cramping. As with other herbs, antispasmodics each have an affinity to specific areas within the body (e.g., menstrual cramping, urethra cramping, leg cramps, tense muscle shoulders, etc).

Anti-thelmintic herbs are used to combat parasitical worms in the body. Finding worms within the digestive tract is more common than you would think, even here in the U.S., especially for children who have a tendency to put things in their mouths that are not food products.

Astringent herbs tighten and tone tissues. Tightening and toning tissues can also help to prevent infection. Think of these for spongy gums, infections of the mucosal membranes such as a sore throat, vaginal infection, ulcers in the digestive tract, urinary tract infections, varicose veins and diarrhea.

Bitters refer to the taste of a plant. The bitter taste creates a cascade of digestive events, from increased salivation to increased HCL in the stomach, to the release of bile and pancreatic enzymes. Bitters are a wonderful way to prestart the digestive process before a meal and ensure the foods you are eating get fully digested. They will also help people who have acid reflux. Most people have no idea that acid reflux is not from too much acid; it is actually from too little. Drinking a cup of warm tea with bitter herbs about 15 minutes before dinner will do wonders.

Cardio tonic herbs are used to support heart and blood vessel function. They have observable beneficial actions on the heart but do not contain cardiac glycosides found in our more dramatic acting plants. Although considered safe, they can interact with some pharmaceutical drugs.

Carminative herbs are used for digestive issues such as bloating and gas. These herbs are often aromatic or strong smell and contain volatile oils. Breastfeeding mothers can often drink teas made with these herbs to help babies with colic.

Cholagogue herbs increase the production and release of bile. Most bitters are cholagogue. As they stimulate bile secretion and peristalsis they may be somewhat laxative in nature. They help to improve hepatic, or liver, function and can increase a person's ability to digest fats.

Circulatory herbs are used for sluggish circulation, like cold hands and feet. They are often added in lesser amounts to formulas to distribute the herbs throughout the body. They are also added to balms or salves to help draw the herbs through the skin and into the blood stream or increase surface circulation.

Demulcent herbs are slimy and mucilaginous in quality. These herbs are used to soothe hot and irritated tissues, like putting aloe gel on a sunburn. Demulcent herbs are also used for a sore throat, digestive ulcers, dry and unproductive coughs, irritated intestines and an irritated urinary tract.

Relaxing diaphoretics are used when a person has a fever, and they feel hot and look hot, but they are not sweating. They may have a red face and be tense or restless. Relaxing diaphoretic herbs may increase peripheral (head, hands, and feet) circulation to release the exterior and open the pores, kind of opening the windows in a hot house. Some relaxing diaphoretic herbs also specifically relieve the aches and pains associated with fevers.

Stimulating diaphoretics are used when a person has a fever, but they feel chilled and are shivering. The spicy herbs support the body's desire to increase our internal temperature.

Diffusive herbs break up stuck energy and move it throughout the body. Have you ever eaten a hot pepper and felt the heat in your toes and fingers? That is diffusive. Diffusive herbs are often used for stagnant digestion (like if you feel you have a bowling ball in your stomach after eating) and are often added in small quantities to formulas.

Diuretic herbs increase urine output. They can be used to lower blood pressure, resolve damp conditions in the body (edema) or for infections of the urinary system. They generally work best as a lukewarm tea.

Emmenagogue herbs promote menstruation and are used for irregular or stagnant menstruation. Emmenagogue herbs should be avoided in pregnancy.

Relaxing expectorants are often demulcent (soothing), antitussive (cough reliever) and anti-inflammatory. They soothe bronchial tissues (via a reflexive action) and can move dry stuck mucus. Often times these herbs are cooling.

Stimulating expectorants motivate mucus expulsion, especially for stuffy conditions. Have you even eaten spicy mustard or wasabi (horseradish) and then felt your sinuses drain? That is a stimulating expectorant. At times these are warming in nature and can work by irritating the bronchial tissues. These herbs often have volatile oils and alkaloids.

Immunomodulating herbs build and strengthen the immune system. They are generally used for people who get sick all the time with colds and the flu or have other symptoms of immune system dysfunction such as seasonal allergies, environmental allergies, food intolerances, and autoimmunity problems. Think of these as deeply nourishing food and herbs for the immune system.

Immunostimulant herbs boost the immune system in the short term. These herbs are generally not taken in the long term and should not be used to compensate for a weakened and unhealthy immune system.

Laxative herbs increase bowel movements. They can range from supportive and gentle to more purgative in effect. Some laxative herbs increase peristalsis (muscle contraction) of the bowels, others may provide lubrication. In general, it is always good to start with the most gentle and work up. It is imperative not to rely on stimulating or cathartic laxatives to move the bowels since they can easily create dependency. Use of laxative herbs may cause griping or pain and so they are usually used in a formula to offset those effects. Using these herbs for

more than ten consecutive days may cause dependency.

Lymphatic herbs are a specialized type of alterative. Lymphatic herbs move congested lymph and can be used to shrink swollen lymph glands and dissolve benign cysts.

Relaxing nervines relax the nervous system. Several of these were mentioned in the chapter on behavioral disorders. Some herbs are merely calming; others can have a more overt sedative effect to promote sleep.

Stimulating nervine herbs stimulate the nervous system. This may be through direct stimulation, such as caffeine from tea or coffee, or stimulating nervine herbs may promote circulation or have a diffusive effect that wakes up the nervous system.

Trophorestorative herbs bring balance to a particular organ or system in a person whether that function is excess or deficient.

Tonic is a troublesome word in the herbal arena as this term is used differently between western and eastern herbal systems. Some western herbalists use it to describe alterative, eliminating or draining herbs. They also might use it to describe herbs that strengthen a system. Raspberry leaf is considered to be toning to the uterus. Dandelion root tones the digestive system. Eastern herbal traditions use the term tonic to describe herbs that are building and nourishing. These herbs tend to be sweet in taste and are taken over a long time by people who have signs of deficiency.

Vulnerary herbs are used to heal wounds. They can be used for external wounds on the skin, or internal wounds such as ulcers or hemorrhoids.

ESSENTIAL OILS

Scientists have been studying the use of essential oils for the treatment of a variety of psychiatric disorders as far back as the 1920's. These studies were published in non-peer reviewed journals and as a result the scientific accuracy could not be confirmed (Lis-Balchin, 2006). Even without verification, the studies were able to determine which essential oils were sedating and which were stimulating. The data collected in these studies provided concrete proof that the constituents in certain essential oils will interfere with the synaptic levels of the neurotransmitter mechanisms. Which I take to mean that they will slow down the over-firing of the synaptic responses that occur when one is anxious. The following essential oils have been utilized to treat a variety of mental, emotional, and behavioral disorders.

Bergamot (*Citrus bergamia*) – Antidepressant, calming, relaxing, sedative

Chamomile – Roman (*Chamaemelum nobile*) – Analgesic, hypnotic, sedative

Geranium (*Pelargonium graveolens*) – Analgesic, antidepressant, uplifting

Jasmine (*Jasminum grandiflorum*) – Antidepressant, euphoric, stimulating, relaxing

Juniper (*Juniperus communis*) – Analgesic, mentally clearing

Lavender (*Lavandula angustifolia*) – Antidepressant, calming, sedative, hypnotic, anti-anxiety

Lemon (*Citrus limonum*) – Mentally stimulating, reviving

Mandarin (*Citrus deliciosa*) – Sedative, uplifting

Marjoram (*Organum majorana*) – Analgesic, comforting, sedating, anti-anxiety

Melissa (*Melissa officinalis*) – Anti-anxiety, calming, sedative, uplifting, stimulating

Neroli (*Neroli bigarade*) – Sedative, uplifting

Patchouli (*Pogostemon cabin*) – Calming, sedating, uplifting

Rose – Egypt (*Rosa damascena*) – Antidepressant, relaxing, soothing, uplifting, sedative

Rosemary (*Rosmarinus officinalis*) – Anti-anxiety, stimulating, clarifying, analgesic

Sage (*Salvia officinalis*) – Nerve tonic

Spearmint (*Mentha spicata*) – Stimulating, analgesic

Vetiver (*Vetivera zizanoides*) – Calming, nerve tonic, uplifting, sedative

Ylang Ylang (*Cananga odourata*) – Analgesic, relaxing

With the use of essential oils on the rise by individuals who have received no formal education on the use of or even an understanding of the potency of these volatile oils, it is both extremely important and my responsibility as a holistic practitioner to share the importance of using **certified organic** essential oils. The potency of essential oils is equal to 30 times that of a cup of herbal tea. Imagine, when using non-organic oils, putting that concentration of herbicides or pesticides on or in your body or your child's body. Never fall for the trademarks out there that claim "certified therapeutic grade" which has no scientific bearing on essential oil quality. And never take the work of a salesperson (or MLM associate) when it comes to the quality of the oils they are selling. If the label says anything other than ***ORGANIC – walk away!***

Chapter 13

How to Use Natural Therapies

Though most herbs are safe for use by anyone, it is always better to contact a professional herbalist, holistic practitioner or naturopath who is knowledgeable in the use and preparation of herbs and herbal therapies. Take the time to research the herbs you are considering using. Look at a minimum of three diverse sources of information. Like medical doctors, each herbalist has their own opinion on which herbs work best in each situation. When looking for reliable sources of information on herbs and herbal formulas, look for books or articles written by trained herbalists. Many professional herbalists belong to the American Herbalist Guild (AHG). Prior to becoming a member of the AHG, an herbalist must provide documented information regarding their education and/or training.

Unlike many medical doctors, most holistic practitioners will spend a minimum of one hour with you on your first visit. A practitioner that is genuinely concerned about your health and wellness should take the time to get to know you and your individual lifestyle. Never be afraid to ask your practitioner about their education and/or training.

There are many ways that herbs and herbal formulas can be made. Most people have heard of herbal teas.

Infusion –Infusions are used internally and/or externally to relieve a wide variety of ailments. An infusion is a water and herb combination – similar to a tea – most often made when using the leaves, buds, fruits, or flowers of the herbs. Infusions can be made with dried, fresh, or powdered herbs. To make an infusion, bring one cup of water to a boil in a stainless steel, glass or ceramic teapot or saucepan. When the water is boiling, remove the pot from the heat and add about one teaspoon of your herb of choice for each cup of water. Place the lid on the pot and allow the herbs too steep for 5-10 minutes. Strain the herbs and enjoy.

If you are drinking herbal infusions for an acute condition, in most cases you can enjoy a cup of tea every hour until symptoms are relieved. If you are drinking herbal infusions for a chronic condition, the dose may be a cup of tea, two or three times a day.

Decoction –A decoction is also a water and herb combination that is made when the herbs in use are roots, seeds, nuts, and barks. Decoctions are often stronger than infusions and can also be used internally and/or externally. To make a decoction, add the herbs to the water in the stainless steel, glass or ceramic pot and bring to a slow boil. Cover and simmer the mixture for 15-20 minutes or longer if making a larger quantity of tea. Remove the pot from the heat, leaving the lid on, and allow it to steep for another 5-10 minutes. Strain and enjoy.

If possible, drink your infusion or decoction without adding a sweetener. If you are totally unable to get past the taste, and some herbs can taste pretty bad, you can add herbs like peppermint or spearmint during the steeping stage to improve the flavor. You can also add honey, agave, or stevia to your tea to sweeten it up a bit. Make every effort to stay away from white sugar, beet sugar, or corn syrup products.

If straining leaves, bark and roots seems a bit overwhelming, or you are worried you will be unable to get all the small parts out, try placing your herbs in a mesh tea ball or using a coffee/tea infuser. The infusers work better when using the leaves and flowers of the herbs. Infusions and decoctions can be kept in the refrigerator up to three days.

Capsules – Capsules contain the ground up or powdered form of the dried herbs and are usually less potent than tinctures or teas. Using capsules is a way to avoid the often strong taste of whole herbs; however, it is often the taste that helps the plant transfer its medicinal qualities to you. Unless you have incredibly good digestion, you are probably not receiving the optimal benefits of the herbs you are taking in capsule form. If you intend to purchase your herbs in prepared form from the local health food store, take note regarding whether the capsules are made from the whole herb or whether the formula has been "standardized." You can tell this by reading the front of the label. If the herbal product has been standardized, that means that a scientist somewhere has identified one or two constituents (plant active ingredients), concentrated these ingredients, and is selling the herbal product in that form. If you are wondering why a company would do that, well it is the money again. Whole plants cannot be patented. Brands such as Traditional Medicinals (teas), Herb Pharm, Gaia Herbs, Mountain Rose Herbs, Rainbow Light Nutritional Systems, New Chapter, and Barlean's Organic Oils are high quality, whole herb products, from companies that stress the importance of ethics in their business practices. Make sure your studies include potential contraindications (when you must avoid taking them) on any herbs you plan to include in your daily routine or that of your child. Again, keep in mind that commercially prepared products list recommended dosage specific to a 150 lb. adult. Adjust the dosage as needed.

Electuary –An electuary is an old fashioned way of taking unpleasant tasting herbs to children. Take a small amount of powdered herb (remember the average capsule contains 1/8 to 1/4 teaspoon of powdered herbs) and mix it with honey, peanut butter, agave, or maple syrup until it reaches a soft consistency.

Candy Balls –Herbal candy balls can be used by anyone of any age for any ailment or disorder. If you make these candy balls, your kids will not even know they are getting a full dose of herbs. All you need are about one cup of sesame or almond butter and a half-cup of honey or agave syrup. Mix these ingredients together until a smooth paste forms. You can add up to eight tablespoons of powdered herbs, bee pollen, Spirulina, chlorella, unsweetened coconut, chopped fruit, ground nuts or carob chips. Mix all the ingredients well, adjusting flavors to taste. Roll into balls and finish by rolling in the unsweetened coconut or some powdered slippery elm. Eat and enjoy. Children can eat one or two of these herbal candy balls up to three times a day. When you are not giving the candy balls to your children, keep them up out of their reach. The candy balls do not need to be refrigerated, however, if it is really warm, you may want to store them to maintain freshness.

Extracts –An extract is a combination of herbs, dried, fresh, or powdered, with a solvent such as grain alcohol, grape brandy, vegetable glycerin, water, and/or vinegar. Many herbal preparations are labeled as extracts when they are actually tinctures. The difference is in the preparation method. Though anyone can make an extract or tincture for their own personal use, I would advise contacting a certified herbalist for correct guidelines on the proper preparation or for a high quality commercial herbal brand.

Smoothies –What child does not like a fruit smoothie? Powdered herbs can be added to any smoothie recipe with minor change in the overall flavor. Try using soy, almond, coconut, goat, or organic milk along with a superior quality yogurt and fresh or frozen fruit. Add about one teaspoon of powdered herbs per serving. Blend until smooth and creamy. Pour and enjoy.

Pills – Pills are made with dried, ground herbs. They are extremely easy to make. Mix the powdered herbs with a little honey until it reaches a paste-like consistency. Roll this mixture into small BB sized balls. Dry for 24-48 hours prior to using. The pills can be swallowed whole, chewed up, or crushed and mixed into applesauce or oatmeal.

So how much of the herbal preparation should you give to your child? A good practitioner will explain to you that in using over the counter medications or herbal formulas – unless specified for children – the dosage instructions are given for a 150 lb. person. Dosages are better adjusted according to the weight of the person taking the formula. If you are seeing an herbalist or holistic practitioner, they will give you the correct guidelines. If not, use the 150 lbs. as a starting point. If you child weighs 50 lbs., you will give your child one-third of the dosage recommended on the bottle. Because each person is an individual and their bodies will react differently to each formula, start with the lowest dosage and work from there. If you are taking more than one herb you have not taken before, do not take them at the same time the first few times you take them. If your body is going to react to the herbs, you need to know which herb you took and when so you can advise your practitioner.

On most herbal tincture remedies, the dosage is listed by drops. The dropper on a 1-ounce bottle holds approximately 30-40 drops. The dropper on a 2-ounce bottle holds approximately 40-50 drops and the dropper on a 4-ounce bottle holds approximately 60-70 drops. A 1-ounce bottle holds 30ml, 1 ounce, or about thirty droppers full.

When should you take your herbs? If possible, try taking your herbs at least 15-30 minutes before you eat or 2 hours after (unless you are using herbs to aid digestion). If you take the herbs at the same time as you eat, the herbs are going to have to compete with the food you ate for digestion and absorption.

The goal of using herbal formulas is to assist the body in its attempt to restore balance. So how long should you take herbal formulas? A general rule is 30 days for each year the individual has experienced the symptoms. Improvements should be noticeable in 1-4 weeks. If you have not observed any improvement in this length of time, discontinue use and see your herbalist or holistic practitioner for a reformulation of the remedy. Continue using the herbal remedy for 1-2 weeks after the symptoms have subsided to ensure that balance has been restored to the body.

Chapter 14
Adverse Reactions

The most common side effect using plant medicine is the possibility of an allergic reaction for people known to have hay fever or other outdoor allergies. If you experience any side effects, such as rash, headache, dizziness or stomach upset, discontinue use, and contact your herbalist or practitioner.

As with any medical treatments, contact your child's medical/herbal practitioner before beginning any program.

Contraindications by body/glandular system

For children that may currently be receiving treatment for disorders of any of the following body/glandular systems, contact a medical professional before taking any of the below listed herbs.

NEUROENDOCRINE: PITUITARY/LIMBIC "POTENTIATING"

Centella asiatica (Gotu Kola)

Oplopanax horridum (Devil's Club)

NEUROENDOCRINE: THYROID STIMULATING

Centella asiatica (Gotu Kola)

NEUROENDOCRINE: ALDOSTERONE SYNERGISTS

Glycyrrhiza glabra (Licorice)

NEUROENDOCRINE: FLAVIN-MAO-INHIBITING

Eschscholzia californica (California Poppy)

Hypericum perforatum (St. John's Wort)

Gingko biloba (Maidenhair Tree)

METABOLIC: ANABOLIC

Oplopanax horridum (Devil's Club)

METABOLIC: ANTICOAGULANT, "BLOOD THINNING"

Centella asiatica (Gotu kola)

Ginkgo biloba (Maidenhair Tree)

CVS: BRADYCARDIC/HYPOTENSIVE

Crataegus pinnatifita (Hawthorn)

Eschscholzia californica (California Poppy)

Passiflora incarnate (Passionflower)

CVS: HYPERTENSIVE POTENTIAL

Glycyrrhiza glabra (Licorice)

Eleuthero coccussenticosus (Eleuthero)

Rhodiola rosea (Rhodiola)

Herb Specific Problems

Angelica (Angelica archangelica) - Diabetes

Ginkgo biloba (Maidenhair Tree) – Reports indicate that it has been used excessively by students when cramming for tests. Under these misguided uses it may cause headaches.

Lemon Balm (Melissa officinalis) - Hypothyroidism

Periwinkle (Vinca minor) – Cerebral hyperemia * brain tumor * brain injury

St. John's Wort (Hypericum perforatum) - May create photosensitivity to direct sunlight (Studies on cows that ate wild St. John's Wort until the plants were completely gone).

References

Alfs, M. (2003) *300 Herbs -Their Indications and Contraindications*

America's Health Rankings (2023) *ADD/ADHD Treatment – Children – United States*

Aromatherapy for Psychiatric Disorders (2014) *CNS Drugs 20(4)* p.259

Bruno, G., and Presser, A. (2005, November). *Health Supplement Retailer*, Living with Diabetes - Supplements to Make the Job Easier (Part 1)

Camardella, E. (2006, December). *Natural Products Marketplace* - Growing Interest, Growing Bodies

CCHR International (2014). Parents: Get the facts— Know your rights. Retrieved from http://www.cchrint.org/issues/childmentaldisor ders/

Centers for Disease Control and Prevention (2025) *State-based Prevalence of ADHD Diagnosis and Treatment 2016-2019 and 2020-2023*

Chartier, K. (2006, September). *Health Supplement Retailer*. Feed Your Brain

Food and Drug Administration - www.fda.gov

Health A to Z. (2008). Drug Leaflet. Retrieved
from: www.healthatoz.com

Hoffman, D. (2003). Medical Herbalism: The science
and practice of medical herbalism. Rochester,
VT: Inner Traditions

Lis-Balchin, M. (2006). Aromatherapy science: A
guide for healthcare professionals. London:
Pharmaceutical Press

Tenney, L. (1996). *Today's Herbal Health for Children*

US Centers for Disease Control and Prevention -
http://www.cdc.gov/ncbddd/adhd/data.html

US Centers for Disease Control and Prevention. State
Profiles. (2013). Retrieved from
http://www.cdc.gov/ncbddd/adhd/stateprofiles/i
ndex.html

Wingert, P. and Kantrowitz, B. (1997, October).
Newsweek Magazine

Appendix A
Dirty Dozen & Clean 15 List

The fruits and veggies with the MOST pesticides are:

1. Spinach – Spinach and lettuce have lots of surface area for pesticides to cover.

2. Strawberries – Out-of-season, imported strawberries are the most risky.

3. Kale, Collard, & Mustard Greens

4. Grapes

5. Peaches

6. Cherries

7. Nectarines

8. Pears

9. Apples – Be aware that scrubbing and peeling will never get all the pesticides off. The heavy waxing of apples also traps pesticides underneath.

10. Blackberries

11. Blueberries

12. Potatoes, sweet bell peppers, hot peppers, and green beans - Peppers absorb pesticides like a sponge. A high percentage of peppers contain pesticides, and many are imported from countries with looser standards than the US has.

Clean 15 - Fruits and veggies with the Least amount of pesticides are:

1. Pineapple
2. Sweet corn (non-GMO)
3. Avocado
4. Papaya (non-GMO)
5. Sweet Onion
6. Sweet Pea
7. Asparagus
8. Cabbage
9. Watermelon
10. Cauliflower
11. Banana
12. Mango
13. Carrot
14. Mushroom
15. Kiwi

The Environmental Working Group (EWG) has collected Department of Agriculture data every year since 1999. From that data, they have published the Dirty Dozen & Clean 15 list.

Appendix B
Natural Sweetener Conversation Table

Sweetener	1 Cup White Sugar Equals	Liquid	Note
Agave nectar	3/4 cup	Reduce 1/3 total	Lower oven temp by 25°
Barley malt syrup	1 ½ cups	Reduce slightly	
Birch syrup (xylitol)	1 cup		Does not work well in breads or hard candies
Birch syrup	1/2 - 3/4 cup	Reduce slightly	
Brown rice syrup	1 ½ cups	Reduce slightly	Good for hard or crunchy baked goods
Date sugar	2/3 – 1 cup		Burns easily
Honey	1/2 - 3/4 cup	Reduce by 1/4 cup; if no liquid,	Lower oven temperature by 25°

		add 3 T flour for each 1/2 cup of honey	
Maple syrup	3/4 cup	Reduce by 3 T	Add 1/4 t baking soda
Maple sugar	1 cup		Add 1/8 t baking soda
Molasses	1/2 cup		
Rapadura & Coconut sugar	1 cup		
Stevia	1 t	Add 1/8 cup	May need to experiment
Sucanat	1 cup		Add 1/4 t baking soda

About the Author

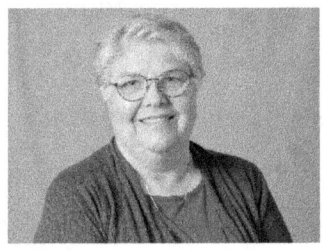

Over 20 years ago, Mary started down a path to learn as much as she could to help her youngest son who had been diagnosed with ADHD. The pressure to medicate him was unreal. No parent or child should be treated that way.

Families deserve better - You deserve better – Your child deserves better

Mary is different than many other authors and practitioners because she has been there. She was a single mom of 3 whose youngest son was labeled with ADHD, at the age of 5, after a 15-minute interview. After being forced to put her son on psychotropic medications, she pursued formal education including two associate's degrees, a Bachelor of Science, and two master's degrees, and a certification in holistic nutrition to support this cause. Mary supports the use of holistic solutions in place of psychotropic medications. She truly desires to provide valuable information, so other parents have real solutions to support their own authentic children in a holistic way.

She is the author of four non-fiction books, Parenting Consciously - Out of the Box Solutions for

Nurturing Your Authentic Child; Recognizing the Greatness in Each Child – Because Learning Differently Doesn't Mean Learning Disabled; Plants vs Pills - Natural Solutions to the Over-Drugging of America's Youth; and un-Broken Children - Removing Labels Restoring Health & Wellness, and as a co-author of the International Best-Seller, My Big Idea Book from Expert Insights Publishing.

Mary is the proud mother of three grown authentic children and grandmother of five. She has lived in several states, including Missouri, Arizona, Alaska, Washington, Colorado, Western North Carolina and currently resides in Virginia with her kitty, MoJo. Her current passion project is to identify several acres where she can design a nature play land, a safe place for today's authentic children, and their parents, to discover their personal connection with nature.

www.ingramcontent.com/pod-product-compliance
Lightning Source LLC
Chambersburg PA
CBHW070353290526
45790CB00004B/1467

* 9 7 8 1 5 0 8 8 4 7 6 4 9 *